Babies in the Cornfield

Stories of Maternal Health and Death from around the World

ANN DAVENPORT

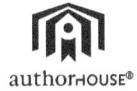

authorHOUSE®

AuthorHouse™
1663 Liberty Drive
Bloomington, IN 47403
www.authorhouse.com
Phone: 1-800-839-8640

First published by AuthorHouse 6/26/2009

ISBN: 978-1-4389-8518-3 (e)
ISBN: 978-1-4389-8517-6 (sc)

Printed in the United States of America
Bloomington, Indiana

This book is printed on acid-free paper.

Acknowledgements

I'd like to express my heartfelt gratitude to all the women who ever helped me to know that being female is an honor and a privilege, starting with my granny Ann, my mother Jean, my cousin Donna, my three sisters and sister-in-law, and all the mothers I have had the honor to attend. Thank you to all the midwives and nurses who taught me that caring for others is an opportunity for growth, especially Marina Alzugaray, Deborah Bossemeyer, Colleen Conroy, Linda Corbet, Debbie Diaz, Sushie Engelbrecht, Elena Esquiche, Jane Ann Fontenot, Frances Ganges, Patricia Gomez, Dian Holzer, Jenna Houston, Martha Hughes, Gloria Iribarne, Barb Kinzie, Marina Lembo, Peg Marshall, Jeanne McDermott, Joan Isabella Paluzzi, Pam Putney, Jemima Rodriguez, Laura Cao Romero, Jan Tritten, Loreto Urmeneta, Claudia Vera, Gilda Vera, Delia Susana Veraguas, and Naoli Vinaver. My gratitude to all the doctors of medicine and other sciences who showed me that you don't need to test your "power-over" people to make changes, and who have become good friends because of their women-centered convictions, especially Robbie Davis-Floyd, Marge Koblinsky, Edgar Necochea, Michel Odent, Harshad Sanghvi, Ilse Santizo, Jeff Smith, Luis Tavara, and Marsden Wagner. My warm regards to my writing mentors at the Johns Hopkins University, including David Everett, Melissa Hendricks, and Ed Perlman. I am blessed to have spiritual midwives who guided me through the birthing of this book; Carol Gaskin (a fantastic editor) and Lynne Butterworth (my doula). I wouldn't have been able to write any of this without the love and support of my favorite midwife and best friend, Gloria Maria Metcalfe. Muchas gracias.

Table of Contents

Introduction

White the life force represents the culture of hope for every human society, it may also give personal meaning to young women who may feel they have no purpose in life except to reproduce themselves. Childbirth gives meaning for everyone around this girl as well: her family, her village or neighbors, and the nurses, midwives, and doctors who care for her all feel relevant and proud when they become involved in this life force.

In his book 'War is a Force That Gives Us Meaning'[1], author and war correspondent Chris Hedges writes about how the force of war also promotes its own culture. He explains, "The enduring attraction of war is this: Even with its destruction and carnage it can give us what we long for in life. It can give us purpose, meaning, a reason for living." His book resonated intensely with me, given what I have come to know of purpose and meaning.

I am a midwife and a nurse. I have seen destruction and carnage from the age of eighteen as a paramedic during the Viet Nam War and later as a midwife working in places from Kosovo to Pakistan. I have also seen pregnancy and childbirth become a magnificent force of life, a force that dares and rejects death, from Mexico to Chile, Uganda to Indonesia, and in thirteen other countries.

Unfortunately, attitudes toward childbirth can progress from respect and awe at this force of nature, to one of suspicion and fear: for don't all forces of nature require management and conquest?

Thus, childbirth becomes something to control. A reason to bring on the technology. Medical science, surgical training, and the hospital industry all search for ways and reasons to control and confront the unpredictable. And in the fight for control, just like in a war, there are winners and losers.

In this book, I'd like to address some of the questions we may face while considering how birth is a force that gives everyone meaning. What is it that makes frightened professionals crave control over a force of nature? How do women who give birth naturally explain their creative power and inner authority to those who prefer anesthesia and major surgery? Why does the business of technology have precedence over the thriftiness of common sense and faith in a natural biological process? How can manipulation of the matriarchal life force have long-term secondary effects on society? And who is making these life and death decisions about pregnancy and childbirth? A hint -- it's not the woman.

I had worked in the United States' dysfunctional health care system for twenty-two years before I bailed out, and into Bolivia, where I began an overseas public health career. For the past fifteen years, I have learned much of other cultures and health customs while I worked on the "front lines," so to speak, with midwives, medical personnel, and women in labor. I have learned how medical management can facilitate the life force or block it with disastrous consequences. And I have learned how each one of us is responsible for the lives of our global neighbors -- whether we like it or not.

Connection, from the micro to the macro, supports our reasons for being. I hope these essays and reflections will help those of us who work with childbearing women to connect to those who are pregnant. I hope they will help people who may never have a baby, yet make public policy, connect to pregnant women and their families. I hope they will help people who study the social and anthropological workings of a society connect to those just trying to survive in it. And finally, I hope that these essays will help those who value the force of life over death connect to those who are striving to survive.

In this book I'll illustrate experiences from nurses, midwives, and a few doctors around the world who do manage to make connections: technology with cultural values, a woman's needs with those of her family or community, and prevention with appropriate intervention. These experiences show, again and again, that the only way to connect with the life force is to value love over fear, and to trust in the power of that love. The modern doctor/ scientist model trusts technology thereby alleviating their own fear of "uncontrollable" forces of nature. The midwife model trusts nature and the life force, to trust a woman's natural ability to give birth, thus to connect everyone involved to the essence of life and love. The medical model focuses on pathology, while the midwifery model focuses on health and well-being.

Judith Pence Rooks says the following about the difference between these two models in her book 'Midwifery and Childbirth in America'[2]:

> "Whereas medicine focuses on the pathologic potential of pregnancy and birth, midwifery focuses on its normalcy and potential for health. Pregnancy, childbirth, and breastfeeding are normal bodily and family functions. That they are susceptible to pathology does not negate their essential normalcy and the importance of the non-medical aspects of these critical processes and events in people's lives. Midwives know about the medical risks, identify complications early, and collaborate with physicians to assure medical care for serious problems. But attention to the medical aspects of these complex processes, while essential, is not sufficient. Midwives focus on each woman as a unique person, in the context of her family and her life. The midwife strives to support the woman in ways that empower her to achieve her own goals and hopes for her pregnancy, birth and baby, and for her role as mother. Midwives believe that women's bodies are well designed for birth and try to protect, support, and avoid interfering with the normal processes of

labor, delivery, and the reuniting of the mother and newborn after their separation at birth."

Through the stories I have included here, a enormous picture begins to emerge, a picture both frustrating and hopeful. Each year, millions of dollars are spent on programs meant to improve maternal and infant mortality, as well as women's overall health, and each year a large percentage of these misspent dollars fail to deliver the desired results. Stories from the very people who are working with pregnant women and their newborns, worldwide, have much to offer in the way of hope and common sense to physicians and policy-makers who need to learn from the midwifery model of care.

Finally, I hope to address the query put forth by anthropologist Emily Martin in her book "The Woman in the Body".[3] She asks, "What would be lost if women were removed from birth?" I have some stories to share that will reveal not only what would be lost, but how and why. The good news is, many people are working very hard to help deny the force of fear that wants to conquer the force of life and birth. Women all around the world know that in our ability to give birth, to bring life into the world, and to nurture that tiny spark of hope -- whether we choose to give birth or not -- is the true force that gives every human meaning.

CHAPTER 1

Who Knew?

I remember the first time I did a vaginal exam on a woman in labor during a "house call" in the mountains of western Bolivia. When I turned my back to wash my hands, she ran out the door, waddled up the hill, and birthed her baby in a dense cornfield. As a midwife, I had been trained to investigate, to prepare. How many centimeters dilated? Is it time to "deliver" the baby? Hot water and warm towels in the room? This was her seventh baby, a baby that would be born at home, without help, and drop onto the waiting sheepskin floor cover just like the first six before him. She didn't need me telling her when it was time to give birth. Her body knew. I was the one who didn't know anything. This rural woman was shamed by me, made nervous by me, and risked her life and her baby's life by running away from me. Some midwife. Some "authority on childbirth."

Those of us who have a university education think we know what's best for those who don't. Thanks to well-meaning, monied people from already-developed rich countries, health care reform is on the agenda everywhere, and should be. But who is writing that agenda? Most likely those same people who were taught inside Institutions of Higher Learning – people who live light years from the only mud-slick road to the health post, where the doctor is out, the pharmacy does not exist, and the next bus to a city with a hospital leaves on Wednesday.

Millions of educated minds strategize and tinker with health policy, from the UN's World Health Organization and the World Bank's Structural Adjustment Policies, to thousands of non-governmental organizations, religious institutions, and tired doctors on track toward their retirement at Ministries of Health or the Centers for Disease Control. Some believe that high-tech interventions are the way to prevent women and babies from dying by the bus-load every day – and that low-tech or even no-tech interventions are old-fashioned or dangerous ideas.

As recently as 1992, for example, Dr. Keith Russell, former president of the American College of Gynecologists and Obstetricians, publicly declared that "Home birth is child abuse in its earliest form" (*Los Angeles Times*). Yet that same year, more than a third of all babies born in the Netherlands came into the world on their mother's own bed at home, with a midwife in attendance. The Netherlands is one of several countries in the world with the very *best* maternal and infant health statistics – all at moderate cost. Meanwhile, the high-tech, high-priced health care in the USA suffers by comparison, sneaking in at only number 17 on that list of maternal and infant health rates.[4]

Intervention alone, whether high-tech or low-tech, won't decrease maternal or infant deaths or diseases. But no intervention is worse! In November of 2006, the United Nations Population Fund wrote in their annual report that horrific gender violence, sometimes perpetrated under the protective justification called "traditional cultural practices" – or religious customs where *no one intervenes* – is widespread and deeply rooted. Rape has become a routine weapon of war, and 80 million girls a year are forcibly married before their eighteenth birthdays, at an age when pregnancy is the leading cause of death for adolescent women.[5] The interventionists among us really do want to step in and do something to diminish disease and save lives.

People with university degrees in medicine, midwifery, or nursing tend to see life, and especially birth, as problematic, however. We who have spent years surrounded by fatality, infirmity, and frailty want to step in and rescue. We are *trained* to rescue. The patient (or in most cases, the body, body part, or disease) morphs into a malfunctioning machine to us – and our goal is a well-working machine. With this goal, intervention becomes the norm, preferably using other machines run by technology-savvy physicians. Dr. Marsden Wagner, in his important work *Pursuing the Birth Machine,*[6] reminds us that the "medical model sees health as the result of external agents (treatments) conquering the ever-chaotic and uncontrollable nature of the body, which tends toward disease. If disease results in spite of the best medical interventions, it becomes the failure of the individual in the medical care system."

Educational institutions teach physicians to believe that they are not only capable of that intervention, but obliged to make it! They also learn to make moral, absolute, and objective judgments about people's lives and about what type of health services those lives should receive. According to the medical model, life is a problem, is risky, and needs management. A telling passage about physicians' self-appointed moral obligation can be found on page one, in the very first paragraph, of the primary medical textbook for gynecologists and obstetricians in the entire world, *Williams Obstetrics.* The authors state unequivocally: "Obstetrics is concerned with the reproduction of a society." On that same page, they emphasize that "...obstetrics strives to analyze and influence the social factors that impinge on reproductive efficiency."[7] Thus we see how doctors are trained to believe they are the engineers of the human condition.

In a non-medical, social/ecological model, life is a solution rather than something to be manipulated and rescued. Dr. Wagner, a perinatologist and public health specialist, reminds us in *Pursuing the Birth Machine* that the most important health statistic in the world is the global mortality rate: 100%. And since we all die, the important thing is to live well. Human beings are part of a vast ecological system, one that includes both the interior and the exterior of the organism we inhabit. It includes our social status, our family and community, our support systems, our spiritual beliefs, our mental state, and the physiological care we give to ourselves and each other.

Ina May Gaskin, traditional midwife extraordinaire, author of *Spiritual Midwifery,* [8] and co-founder of The Farm in Summertown, Tennessee, writes that birth is not just a biological event (anatomical, physiological, and biochemical). It's an event that transforms us due to the mental and spiritual components of pregnancy and childbirth. Indispensable to this view, of course, is that birth *by nature* springs from femininity, intuition, sexuality, and spirituality – qualities not found in a medical model more fascinated by quantifying mechanical factors such as fetal monitor strip printouts.

Pregnancy and childbirth say more than any other life event about the status of women in a society. Attitudes toward pregnancy are far more telling than any laws or a country's educational system. Is the pregnancy wanted? By whom? Is the fertility rate mandated by government policy and rewarded or punished? Does a twelve-year-old child bride have a choice about starting a family? Does a woman pregnant for the twelfth time have a choice about terminating that pregnancy or obtaining contraceptives? Are women treated like cattle in a barn or parts on an assembly line during their hospitalized labor, or simply like sick patients? Is there any reason to believe women's experiences if they are unable to produce scientific evidence to support that experience?

Anthropologists have observed that people's belief systems underlie all fundamental practices in all cultures, particularly the rituals and taboos dealing with mating, birth, and death. Modern medicine (especially obstetrics) has emerged as the new and *competing* belief system, with its own set of taboos, rituals, and mysteries – belief systems that are, in a way, the hallmarks of a competing religion.[9]

I don't want this book to leave the reader with the idea that there is no place for medical technology for saving lives, or that all cultural ritual is always a good thing (think female genital mutilation!). The miracles of modern medical technology and tech-savvy doctors saved my life when I had appendicitis and after a car accident. Yet, although technology has indeed saved the lives of many babies and mothers, we must remember that the most important factors for the decrease in maternal mortality (death) and morbidity (illness) rates are not medical but social.[10] These factors include: educating girls, better nutrition, hygienic practices by doctors, and contraception.

The medical model applied to childbirth, and thus applied to public health programs and policy, focuses on curing disease and using technology to do it. In the 1980s, Eastern European countries had much higher infant death rates than Western European countries. The doctors in charge at the Ministries of Health demanded more funds from the World Health Organization (WHO) for neonatal intensive care units and better machines in those units. The WHO physicians pointed out that the majority of their public prenatal clinics still lacked basic, low-tech supplies like stethoscopes or blood pressure cuffs, and that most maternity hospitals didn't even have Ambu bags or oxygen tanks for basic resuscitation.

Whenever we train doctors and midwives in Emergency Obstetric Care in developing countries (sponsored by WHO and the Johns Hopkins Program for International Education in Gynecology and Obstetrics[11]), the first thing the professional participants usually want to know is: When do we have the class on ultrasound or fetal monitoring machines? They are always surprised when we focus on life-saving skills using our five senses, our hands, our stethoscopes and fetoscopes, simple drugs, and straightforward low-tech interventions that prevent complications and save lives.

In general, appropriate technology should be simple, inexpensive, consumer-friendly, non-invasive, and acceptable to the culture and community. In his book about marketing social behavior changes to influence health,[12] Alan Andreason insists that "...the number one feature for influencing healthy behavior is that *consumer acceptance* [not the doctor's, the midwife's or the nurse's acceptance] *is the bottom line.*" Not only must social programs be cost effective, all strategies must begin with the client in mind. Andreason also reminds us to recognize and identify competition and factor that into any public health policy. The most obvious competition to a normal, healthy pregnancy and birth remains cultural ritual and social values – those of the customer *and* those of the medical professionals. An example: the pregnant woman has the common sense and physical need to give birth in an upright position. The doctor is trained to attend a birth with the woman flat on her back, with his comfort in mind, not hers. Who wins this competition? Cost effectiveness in this case means making the woman give birth in an unnatural position.

Another stark example of this competition between customer and medical professionals concerns the caste system in Nepal and India. Only one caste handles blood, and that caste does not include the educated doctor, nurse, or midwife. Health professionals may attend births (that naturally involve blood) only because they use plastic aprons, gloves, and protective eye barriers to prevent the blood from touching them or vice versa. I discovered this when I spent a week in a small town in western Nepal conducting a follow-up visit for a group of midwives who had attended our training in Katmandu earlier that month. I observed a midwife, one of our students, attending a birth with good infection-prevention techniques, providing care and attention, and giving emotional support to the mother. The midwife received the wet little life into her gloved hands, tied and cut the cord, and then passed the crying naked newborn into the waiting naked hands of...the cleaning lady! The bare-handed cleaning lady carried the newly born babe to the sink in the corner of the room, held him under the faucet to wash off the blood, dried him off, wrapped him in a towel, and handed him back to the midwife, who then handed the howling infant back to the mother.

"Wait a minute," I said to this recently re-educated professional. "What is all this about handing a newborn to the cleaning lady and her washing him under a sink? I thought we practiced this in class! *You* are to dry and examine the baby, to make sure it's breathing, and to hand it immediately to the mother to maintain warmth, right?"

Nepalese have a sweet way of bouncing their head from side to side, which can either mean "yes" or "no" depending on the situation. The midwife said to me, "That is true" (bobbing head movement). "However, neither I nor the mother belongs to the caste that touches blood on the newborn. If the mother touches him before he is cleaned, she will not only affect her karma, but that of her newborn son. The cleaning lady is the person who can touch the blood and clean off the baby for the mother." My medical-model mind told me to insist on the Right Way to do things. My common sense and social-model self told me not to even attempt to change a 5,000-year-old cultural value. So, we trained the cleaning lady in immediate newborn care. And even though we had no scientific evidence to support this change in procedure, we did it because we are women with common sense who wanted healthy babies and mothers.

Health procedures and policy cannot be isolated from the larger socio-economic context in which they occur. *Poverty* – not cultural ceremony or medical ritual – contributes to poor health, and poor health contributes to poverty. Anthropologist Joan E. Paluzzi succinctly outlines in *Unhealthy Health Policy*[13] the reasons why the World Bank's structural adjustment policies have *worsened* the quality of life among the world's poorest people: They focus interventions and funding on single-cause/single-intervention programs (for example, HIV prevention funding that denies sex education). The disconnection of policies and programs from real people and real poverty has helped to increase the number of poor people suffering from interconnected health problems.

It may seem like common sense to you and me to ask a person what she wants before we go about giving her what we think she needs. Leave it to the anthropologists, sociologists, and women birthing in cornfields to point out this obvious fact to us. In this book I'd like to discuss experiences from midwives and a few doctors around the world who manage to make the essential connections – balancing technology with cultural values, women's needs with well-intentioned interventions – and who can point the way toward common sense preventive measures and health policies that work.

Pregnant Pause

I will insert little pauses between some chapters, dear reader, because I believe pauses may be used to rest, to reflect, and to provide us with clues with which we may discern subtext or even unconscious content about what we're reading.

For midwives, labor and childbirth is divided into four stages, the first is labor, the second is pushing; the third stage is the birth of the placenta, and the fourth stage is immediate postpartum. In the natural course of labor we often have a lull, or quiet period when the hard contractions have past, the cervix is fully dilated and the woman's body seems to "take a break". This stage is sometimes called "the pregnant pause" because it's a time for the mother to rest and drink liquids and catch her breath – even sleep sometimes – before the Big Push.

I have crafted these pauses with the intent of amplifying or illuminating some points in the text – or sometimes not. Sometimes they are just sprinkled in like a little extra condiment. Use them however you like: to stimulate conversation or reflection, to read while you're between patients or visitors, or while taking a breath before the next chapter.

Here is the first one. Enjoy your pause.

The traditional midwife

Traditional midwives have been an integral part of African medicine for centuries. This is not only because African people still love and fear the spirits, but also because a great number of the South African population do not have access to existing health services."

From *Curationis,* 1997 Mar; 20(1):15-20. Troskie, T.R.,
"The Importance of Traditional Midwives in the Delivery
of Health Care in the Republic of South Africa."

If you do a "Google" search for traditional midwives,
you will get over 861,000 entries...and counting.

CHAPTER 2

What is Maternal Mortality?

Peg Marshall, a certified nurse midwife and our visiting professor from Washington, D.C., walked into our classroom in Lima, Peru, loaded down with posters and papers. She faced our group of twenty doctors and midwives from six Latin American countries. We had gathered together for a week-long workshop about World Health Organization recommendations for reducing maternal death. A sad look on her face caught our attention, and she asked us if we'd heard the tragic news.

"I'm sorry I'm a little late," she said, dropping the papers on her desk, "but I wanted to hear the whole story. It was awful. Didn't any of you hear about the terrible plane crash here in Lima this morning?" None of us had heard anything. "What happened?" "Where was it?" asked a few participants.

"It was one of those big jumbo jets that hold about seven hundred passengers," she said. "All the crew, the pilots – everyone on board was killed. The plane took off from the airport here in Lima and it was out over the Pacific when the engines caught on fire."

We stared at her in disbelief and horror as her hand swept through the air, imitating the arc of the doomed aircraft.

"They made a wide turn to come back to land, and the plane exploded on impact as it reached the ground, killing hundreds in the housing area near the airport. They estimate about fourteen hundred people dead."

Some participants burst out with cries of anger. "No!" Others couldn't speak.

"Yes," Peg calmly replied after a moment. "The most tragic part is that all aboard were pregnant, or were women who had just given birth – all the passengers, even the crew and the pilots. Everyone killed on the ground was pregnant too, or new mothers. Horrible." She shook her head and sighed.

"What?" Her statement stopped us cold. Many of us spoke simultaneously. "All pregnant? How can that be? How do they know? What are you talking about?"

"Amazing, isn't it?" Peg asked. She slowly looked around the room. She leaned forward on her desk and continued in a strong voice. "We are horrified and speechless when we hear that 1,420 women died today in a senseless and preventable accident. Yet when we hear those same numbers as daily maternal deaths, they don't have the same impact. When the World Health Organization estimates that 515,000 women die every year from complications due to pregnancy and childbirth, we think, 'Gee, that's sad.' But those numbers don't have the same emotional impact they did just now, when I said that over fourteen hundred women died *today*. And another 1,420 will die tomorrow, and the next day, and the next."

We stared at her, not knowing what to think.

"Of course there was no plane crash to cause these deaths," she said. "And there was also no news story, no TV cameras, no public outcry, and no congressional demand for an investigation for these very real deaths. Nothing. And that's the *real* tragedy."

I heard that classroom example in Lima in 1996, when the World Health Organization estimated that 515,000 women died every year from complications due to pregnancy or childbirth. The latest statistics from the WHO, for 2005, show no improvement. Worldwide maternal deaths (termed maternal mortality) are estimated to be around 560,000 per year. That means about 1,500 women die *every day* from complications because they were pregnant or giving birth or just had a baby. These deaths are almost equally divided between countries in Africa (251,000) and Asia (253,000). Only four per cent of worldwide maternal deaths (22,000) occur in Latin America and the Caribbean, and less than one per cent (2,500) in the more developed regions of the world.[14]

Events like civil war, along with poverty, ignorance, fear, or traditional practices all contribute to the high rates of maternal death and disability. Other contributors to maternal death include the ability to recognize danger signs and arrive at a hospital. Many women don't know the danger signs that warn of potentially fatal complications, like headache and blurred vision, vaginal bleeding, fever, or prolonged labor. Women and their families in rural areas around the world know that no transportation exists at night to get to a hospital, even if they do recognize danger signs or – worse yet and more common – no hospital is available in their province. Women in rural Afghanistan, Iraq, Indonesia, Yemen, or Sudan, for example, don't dare travel at night, grunting with labor pains or not, because their culture forbids it.

If a woman in labor does make it to a hospital in a developing country, life-saving drugs may not be available for her in case of an emergency. An anesthesiologist or a surgeon may not be on staff in that hospital. The blood bank or transfusion capability may not exist, and probably an operating room with adequate supplies is not available in case she needs a Cesarean section. In government-funded public hospitals around the world, distribution of equipment, supplies, drugs, and professional staff depends on money and motive – factors that sometimes just don't exist. Many women die during pregnancy or childbirth due to neglect, bad health, no funds, no facilities, no well-trained professionals, no supplies, and no national health policy that prioritizes maternal infant care based on the latest scientific evidence or "Best Practices" recommended by that evidence. They die needlessly.

Many women refuse to go to the hospital for many reasons, but mostly because the hospital is where you go to die, not to give birth. In Guatemala, for example, during their thirty-six-year civil war, a woman took her life in her hands if she dared leave her village to go to the hospital, in labor or not. From 1960 to 1990, more than 200,000 people died in Guatemala (the majority indigenous peoples),[15] and more than one million fled the country. It didn't matter whether that escaping woman was pregnant, had just had a baby, or was in labor. Her safest bet was to give birth at home, with the time-honored assistance of her neighborhood traditional midwife – the *comadrona*. This same scenario takes place today in Afghanistan, Iraq, the Democratic Republic of Congo, Sudan, Somalia, and other places where trust and fear become matters of life and death.

At the end of our class in Lima, Peg Marshall talked about other public health statistics, and we investigated the many reasons why a woman may or may not safely survive her pregnancy and childbirth. Violence against women seemed to be the main theme through all the stories. Even in the USA, land of private and expensive health care, of top-flight doctors and high-tech life-saving interventions, women continue to die during their pregnancies. But they don't usually die from any of the five principle causes of global maternal mortality, which are hemorrhage, infection, obstructed labor, eclampsia (convulsions), and embolism. As we'll see in the next chapter, women in the richest country in the world die from something much more sinister and mysterious. And preventable.

Pregnant Pause

Essential Obstetric Care (EOC) Guidelines Defined by the World Health Organization

The WHO defines a "skilled attendant" as a university-trained health provider (nurse, midwife, or physician) who can care for a woman during her labor, birth, and postpartum, and her newborn. It helps if these attendants are supported by an infrastructure that provides **Basic Emergency Obstetric Care.** This means their health facility needs to have the following things in place to be of any help to anyone:

Basic EOC (This means the first level of care – the Health Post or Community Clinic):

- Basic intravenous medications to prevent infection, convulsions, and hemorrhage: ampicillin, gentomycin, magnesium sulfate, and oxytocin, along with basic intravenous (IV) solutions like normal saline or dextrose.
- Skilled staff who know how to manually remove a stuck placenta, placental pieces, or retained pieces from a spontaneous or provoked abortion.
- Basic adult resuscitation equipment and the knowledge for using that equipment (bag and mask, oxygen, suction, IVs)
- Newborn resuscitation equipment and staff know-how (bag and mask, oxygen, suction)
- Knowledge about how to keep a premature baby warm 24 hours a day (the "kangaroo method" of skin-to-skin contact with the mother or other)
- Probably the most important: **Transportation availability 24/7 to a referral hospital**

Comprehensive EOC (sometimes known as "the Referral Hospital"):

- All the above, PLUS...
- Surgical resolution of problems (which means an operating room with skilled staff, anesthesia, oxygen, and sterile equipment)
- Blood bank and laboratory 24/7
- Cardiopulmonary resuscitation of adult or newborn that includes all the above, PLUS intubation skill and equipment, X-ray capabilities, ventilation machines, and cardiac drugs
- Fluid and nutrition management (feeding tubes, special formulas, or IV solutions)
- Thermal regulation for premature babies that involves incubators, oxygen, and bilirubin lights

NONE of the above services are available to about a million pregnant women around the world. Everyone agrees these services should exist, but they do not. Yet, amazingly, people continue to make love and make babies (the best case scenario, ruling out rape) and turn to their village midwife for care, as they have for millions of years.

CHAPTER 3

Do Mothers Count?

Washington Post (AP) November 12, 2004. Scott
Peterson, 32, was convicted today of murdering his
pregnant wife and dumping her body in San Francisco
Bay in what prosecutors in the case portrayed as
a cold-blooded attempt to escape marriage and
fatherhood for the bachelor life. Laci Peterson, a
27-year-old substitute teacher, was eight months
pregnant when she vanished around Christmas
Eve 2002. Four months later, her headless body and
the remains of her fetus were discovered along the
shoreline about 90 miles from the couple's Modesto
home – not far from where her husband claims he
was fishing alone the day of her disappearance.

The coroner who examined Laci Peterson's body wrote "homicide"
on her death certificate. Nowhere did the death certificate mention
that Laci Peterson had been pregnant at the time of her homicide.
Nowhere did the certificate or any other official record note the
phrase "maternal mortality," nor is the execution of any pregnant
woman recorded as a maternal mortality in any country. That's
because the official definition of maternal mortality used in public

records has no clause that mentions the term murder. Why is this so important? If women's deaths by murder aren't counted as maternal mortalities, then there are no public health incentives to fund interventions to prevent these maternal massacres. And public health programs are all about detection and prevention.

Murder is the leading cause of death for pregnant or recently pregnant women in the United States of America. Just take a minute to think about that sentence. The leading cause of maternal mortality in the richest country in the world is homicide. Murder causes more premature demise of mothers than eclampsia, thrombosis, or anesthesia-related deaths (the other top three causes of maternal death in the US).

University of Maryland nurse-midwife and researcher Cara Krulewitch, Ph.D., examined autopsy results of 214 female homicide victims from 15 to 45 years of age in Washington, D.C., between 1988 and 1996.[16] She found murder to be the most common manner of death for both pregnant and non-pregnant women. Her research team also found that pregnant women were *twice as likely to be murdered as non-pregnant women of the same age.* Other researchers across the US corroborated her study by reviewing hundreds of county morgue archives in their own states. All came to the same conclusion: murdered pregnant women are not counted as maternal mortality because they don't fit the definition for maternal mortality.

The international standard for defining demise is the World Health Organization's recently released tenth revision of their *International Statistical Classification of Diseases and Related Health Problems* (ISCD-10).[17] This classification, used worldwide by Ministries of Health and by the CDC in the United States, excludes murder as a cause for maternal mortality because the WHO defines maternal mortality as "Those deaths related to or aggravated by pregnancy complications, *excluding accidental or incidental causes,* occurring during pregnancy or within forty-two days of termination" (italics mine). Remember that term: "related to"...

If a woman dies from any of these five direct causes – hemorrhage, obstructed labor, eclampsia, embolism, or infection

– related to pregnancy or childbirth as identified by the ISCD-10, her death is classified as a maternal mortality and she is counted as a maternal death. Because murder is not included in the WHO maternal mortality definition, tens of thousands of pregnant women's murders go unrecorded as maternal deaths – even if her pregnancy was the excuse used by her assassin to kill her!

Recent public health research by highly qualified investigators call for the WHO to change their definition of death from "related to pregnancy" and include pregnancy-*associated* deaths. Dr. Virginia Frye writes in an editorial in the *Journal of the American Medical Association* [18] that the definition of "pregnancy-associated death" would include "the death of any woman, from any cause, while she is pregnant – or within one year of termination of pregnancy." This broader definition for deaths *associated with* pregnancy (as opposed to *related to* pregnancy) is particularly relevant for public health officials hoping to find ways to help prevent those deaths.

World Health Organization epidemiologists admit in their published statistical reviews that maternal deaths are under-counted by as much as fifty percent in some countries. *Fifty percent.* And in sixty-two countries, no maternal mortality data are recorded at all! The Gambia was the first country to implement a sisterhood approach to measure maternal mortality rates.[19] By asking the sisters of dead women how and when the death occurred, they found more women could be counted in that country's maternal mortality statistics. Some countries charge a fee to register births or deaths, and there are many, many barriers for managing statistics. But by guesswork and statistical epidemiology, the World Health Organization estimates that around 560,000 women in the world die every year from complications *related to* pregnancy or childbirth – about one death every minute. And these dead women are only those who are counted based on the WHO definition of pregnancy-*related* deaths.

"If dead women are not even counted [as maternal mortality cases], then it seems they do not count. We have an invisible epidemic," said Joy Phumaphi in a September 2004 World Health Organization press release.[20] The WHO declares it wants countries to find new ways to count maternal deaths in order to raise awareness for policy makers, to direct funding toward prenatal care, and to finally make a dent in that one, big global number that has not diminished (has in fact increased) in spite of almost two decades of their Safe Motherhood policies and programs: *560,000*.

Yet even the official WHO figures for maternal deaths leave out important facts about the circumstances surrounding those deaths. Those figures do not reveal any background information associated with when, how, or why mothers die – information that could have been useful in preventing their deaths. We know that the four principle pregnancy-related direct causes of maternal mortality are hemorrhage, obstructed labor, infection, and eclampsia. But let's consider the background information in the following true stories, and determine if the cause of death was only *related to* the pregnancy, or *associated with* a cause that, if it had received the appropriate intervention, might have prevented a maternal death. The definitions are from the ISCD-10.

Hemorrhage, n. The escape of large quantities of blood; copious or profuse bleeding.

Nicaragua, 2003. A brown-eyed little girl became the center of a controversy that made headlines throughout Latin America. This nine-year-old compromised the Catholic Church and the Archbishop of Nicaragua, and prompted the resignation of the Nicaraguan Minister of Health.

A twenty-two-year-old man raped his nine-year-old niece. She became pregnant, just after having experienced her very first menstrual period. The family physician declared her little fourth-grade body too young to carry the child to term and said both "mother and child" would probably die. The Catholic Church dispatched an army of God's representatives to all media outlets in all Central American countries, decrying the proposed abortion for the nine-year-old as an act of murder, and pleading for the faithful to pray for her and her unborn child. The Bishop of Managua announced that anyone involved in the abortion would be excommunicated – including the girl herself, who had received her First Holy Communion only two years earlier. (He never mentioned ex-communication for the uncle.)

Dr. Ana Maria Pizarro, a gynecologist who directs the *Si Mujer* ("Yes Woman") health center in Managua, says a Nicaraguan government study in 1996 estimated 36,000 illegal abortions a year were performed in the country of five million people. "Unsafe, illegal abortions are among the leading causes of death for Nicaraguan women," wrote Dr. Pizarro.[21]

The director of the Bertha Calderon Women's Hospital reported that botched abortions were filling half the obstetrics beds. He complained that much of the hospital budget was being spent to save the lives of young girls who have had an abortion. The University of Leon puts the number of high-risk abortions in Nicaragua at close to 80,000 a year.[22] For a therapeutic abortion (at that time), a panel of three physicians had to meet and determine whether a woman deserved a legal and safe termination of her unwanted pregnancy according to a strict legal code. It was up to the bearer of the burden (the woman herself – or, in this case, the child herself) to find the doctors and get them together for a meeting.

It's much easier to get together conservative Christian pastors and Catholic priests for a meeting, and they dictate who receives family planning methods or sex-education information – and who receives abortions when family planning fails (usually those who can pay private doctors). The highest rates for dead women occur in countries where abortion is illegal,[23] and Nicaragua recently (October 2006) passed a law declaring *all* abortions to be illegal.

If this little girl's mother and aunts hadn't had the resources to obtain a safe manual vacuum aspiration for her (a ten-minute procedure that involves a sterile syringe with a manual suction apparatus), she might have bled to death from a botched abortion. The cause of death would have been recorded as a pregnancy-related hemorrhage on the Ministry of Health's "Classification of Death" certificate.

This classification would have left out important pieces of the story *associated* with her death: the social and financial impact of illegal abortion, rape laws, or religious policies dictating health care in secular societies. This background information could have been registered on a pregnancy-*associated* death certificate – if such a thing existed – and that data could have been used to plan programs (like family planning for adolescents or sex education courses for children, or penalties for uncles who rape nieces) that may have helped prevent future maternal mortalities.

Another example of a WHO pregnancy-related definition for maternal death is obstructed labor. Consider the background information in the following case and determine whether the cause of obstruction was pregnancy-related, or something *associated with* the pregnancy that could have been prevented.

Obstructed labor, n. When the physical activities involved in normal vaginal birth are blocked or hindered by physical causes, such as placenta previa or fetal malposition.

Jeff Smith, an obstetrician who has worked for more than three years in Afghanistan, helps the Ministry of Health to plan midwifery training programs in the country. The Malalai Maternity Hospital, the largest maternity hospital in Kabul and the country, serves as an important clinical training site for midwives and doctors. Between forty and sixty births take place a day in this hospital, which now – thanks to many NGO interventions – has a fully functioning operating room, anesthesia capabilities, a blood bank, sterile equipment, and a well-stocked pharmacy. The staff of midwives, nurses, physicians, and technical crew are all well trained and dedicated. "The problem," says Smith, "is that many women here have no self-worth."

"Time and time again," he says, "I have seen patients refuse to make a decision about their own health or their fetus. If the baby is a transverse lie [sideways in the womb and not head down], there is no way that baby is going to get out without a cesarean. Yet the majority of women refuse an operation. They say they cannot make that decision – it's up to their husbands."

Smith says the staff will always ask for the husband to come in. The woman then admits she does not want to be "cut open" under any circumstances, because that would mean a violation of her body – which could be an excuse for her husband to desert her and "his" children. Smith's Muslim friends say that some misinterpretations of the Qur'an inform believers they will spend eternity in the body with which they enter heaven at the time of death. If that body is missing a leg, an eye, or is cut open, that's how they will spend eternity – forever flawed.

"The other women physicians are educated," says Smith. "They try to talk with the patient. Rarely we succeed and have a good outcome. Most of the time the husband just takes her home to die. It's damn frustrating."

Obstructed labor is registered as the pregnancy-related cause of a maternal death, but that does not tell the whole story. A pregnancy-*associated* definition, if one existed, might include other elements, such as misinterpretation of the Qur'an or fear of abandonment. This definition could be useful for policy makers who need information to direct funds toward programs that might prevent those deaths: an education campaign by mullahs about the passages in the Qur'an that clarify a husband's obligation to his wife and children, or a social security system that protects abandoned mothers and children from financial destitution, for example.

Eclampsia, n. Convulsions late in pregnancy in a woman affected with pre-eclampsia.

Eclampsia is a straightforward WHO pregnancy-related definition for maternal mortality. This disease is a major killer of young pregnant women, but a pregnancy-related definition does not tell the background story that a pregnancy-*associated* definition might.

Prudence, an 18-year-old recently married woman, pregnant for the first time and happy about her condition, visited her village midwife in the northern rural area of Ghana, a small agricultural country on the Atlantic Coast of Africa. The village midwife noticed swelling of the face, hands, and legs on Prudence, now in her third trimester of pregnancy. She advised Prudence to walk to the health post in the next village to see the nurse about her abnormal condition. Prudence's husband wouldn't be home until the weekend because he worked up in the mountains in the gold mines, and she wanted to wait and go with him to the health post. Prudence's mother and aunts agreed with her; but by the time Saturday rolled around, Prudence was having "fits" (eclampsia-induced convulsions due to high blood pressure). Alarmed, the mother and aunts found a neighbor with a truck willing to take them into the city. They bundled an unconscious Prudence into the back seat of the double-cab and drove the next four hours to the regional hospital in Tema. Prudence suffered two more convulsions during the journey.

It took the truck driver a few minutes to find the entrance to the emergency room, which turned out to be only for non-obstetric crises. The hospital compound covers about three acres, and it took another few minutes to find the entrance to the obstetric ward. Prudence's mother ran into the labor and delivery ward to find some help. She didn't see any nurses or doctors at first – only the cleaning lady.

"The midwives are with women in delivery," said the cleaning lady, and offered to go find someone. About twenty minutes later, a nurse appeared and helped the women place a barely cognizant Prudence onto the only empty bed, which was in the postpartum ward; two patients had squeezed onto another bed with their newborns to make room. Prudence's mother and aunts were told to wait outside.

The nurse went back into the busy delivery room. The two ward nurses, responsible for about forty-five postpartum patients and their newborns, went back to their charting. Prudence went back to "sleep". The other patients went back to their allotted lunch trays. Occasionally Prudence must have continued convulsing, because one of the patients near her bed found a nurse and complained that "The new lady fell from the bed, Sister, and landed on my food tray." A medical resident making his afternoon postpartum rounds noticed Prudence on the floor, apparently sleeping.

"What's going on here, Sister? Let's get this woman on the bed." One. Two. Three – UMPH! The intern read Prudence's chart for more information. The nurses had no time to write down her blood pressure – which was 220/120 the last time they remembered taking it (normal blood pressure is around 120/80). By now it was 3 P.M. and time for shift change and report to the other nurses. Prudence continued convulsing off and on, although the resident had managed to place a urinary catheter into her bladder (to measure the urine output) and an IV into her vein (to give her the magnesium sulfate needed to prevent convulsions). He ordered more medicine and returned to the surgery suite, where he and the only other doctor in the hospital continued operating non-stop into the night.

Prudence did receive her first dose of magnesium sulfate – but no one had time or had bothered to listen to the fetal heart rate. The only anesthesiologist and surgeon on shift were backed up into the night, and, knowing that the only remedy for eclampsia is to get the baby out, they put Prudence on the waiting list behind other emergency C-sections. Prudence was a quiet patient. She just went unnoticed, really, by an understaffed and overworked team of professionals who knew what to do for eclampsia, but just didn't do it.

By the time her husband arrived at the hospital from the mountains, 9 P.M. that night, Prudence and her very first baby were dead. The medical examiner wrote "maternal mortality due to eclampsia" on his governmental form, and added it to the stack of others to send to the capital, Accra, later that month.

Of course, the pregnancy-*related* cause is clear. The pregnancy-*associated* definition may have helped public health planners determine all the reasons for the non-intervention – and this information may have ignited indignation at the ministry level so they'd send more staff to that hospital, or possibly train and equip the village health post nurse to recognize eclampsia and intervene appropriately with drugs until a C-section could be scheduled. A pregnancy-associated review may have focused on interventions that could have detected the pre-eclampsia and prevented the eclampsia, such as weekly blood pressure checks. No one in the village knew what exactly caused Prudence's death; but they all mourned another young woman's passing from their community.

Physicians know how to treat disease and complications; this is what they are trained to do. Pregnancy is not a disease; and most births don't have complications. Complications that can lead to a woman's death or disability may need treatment, but what prompted the complication in the first place? Can those complications be prevented by social or cultural changes? For example, infection is a major cause of maternal mortality and can very easily be treated, with death denied, if diagnosed early. But what's the story behind the infection? What are the pregnancy-*associated* causes of death by infection that could help prevent this very prominent killer?

Infection, n. The establishment of a pathogen in its host after invasion.

Barbara Kinzie, a nurse midwife, has worked in isolated rural villages in Yemen, Egypt, and Eritrea for many years. She was trained in the medical model about what to do when confronted by an infection: detect the culprit organism and knock it out with the right antibiotics. However, she was unprepared for the causes of some of the infections she encountered in the poor women of the Middle East.

"Many women never even made the trip to the hospital in the capital city," explains Barbara. "Those who did arrive came after hours or days of travel. Many would die on the way. Some women traveled with a fever of 40°C. (104°F) ; higher than I ever thought a person could survive. We would treat the infection with antibiotics and do all the right things to bring down the fever. Many, many times the infection was due to an unbelievable amount of herbs and twigs and other concoctions packed inside the woman's vagina after the [home] birth of her baby. It would take hours and a strong stomach to pick out all the debris and various foul-smelling gunk packed into that woman's red, swollen vagina."

While Barbara talked with the mother she would learn that this post-birth practice was important to make a woman's vagina tight again, like it was when she was a virgin, so she would be desirable to her husband. In these very poor African countries, if a woman is abandoned by the husband, and if she has no father to return to, then she might as well be dead. Often, no one will take in her or her baby.

The pregnancy-related cause of death according to the World Health Organization's ISCD-10 manual would be maternal mortality due to infection. The ISCD-10 does not define death due to practices that attempt to assure a tight vagina for a wandering husband.

The World Health Organization has tried some reforms over the years to convince public health officials to find new ways to protect women and children. In September of 2004, the WHO published *Beyond the Numbers – Reviewing Maternal Deaths and Complications to Make Pregnancy Safer.*[24] The authors suggested that by understanding the reasons behind maternal mortality, providers can develop an understanding of why those deaths happened and how similar deaths can be averted. The document also emphasized interventions according to the principle of the Four Delays, and asked policy makers to examine if women risk death due to:

- Delay in recognition that a problem exists;
- Delay in making the decision to access professional health services;
- Delay in accessing services due to barriers such as distance, cost, or socio-cultural restrictions;
- Delay in receiving adequate care, or receiving care that is actually harmful, once they access services.

Beyond the Numbers, however, tends to blame the victim. The delay in recognizing symptoms and diagnosing her complication becomes her burden. This framework also assumes that women have the authority to make decisions about their pregnancies. This is a major complication in most cultures where, after a millennium or more, women have never been allowed to make decisions about anything – particularly about their own reproductive health. Moreover, the framework assumes that a woman or her family should be responsible for transportation, no matter the social or financial cost.

Social injustice; lack of transportation; lack of vitamins, anti-malarial medication, or anti-retroviral medication for HIV; non-use of condoms; or a woman's subservient place in her culture *do not count*, and the WHO falls short when it suggests that health policy be based on definitions of pregnancy-related deaths.

A new system that allows officials to define maternal deaths according to events *associated with* pregnancy, as Dr. Virginia Frye has proposed in the *JAMA* editorial, would flesh out the vital details of the woman's death and illustrate exactly how abuse, poverty, and low status in society contributes to her demise.

The World Health Organization has Safe Motherhood programs that tend to promote recognition of, but *not intervention in,* the social and cultural factors involved in maternal mortality. Death is only the last chapter of a long story that begins with the birth of a female in her community. In many communities around the world:

- A girl fetus is more likely to be aborted.
- Newborn girls are more often killed at birth (infanticide) than are newborn boys when undesired pregnancy occurs and no abortion is available.
- Men and boys are fed first and given the best food, while girls and mothers are fed last, or not at all if there are no leftovers – and the mothers who fixed the food make this decision!
- Girls are usually last to be educated and last to be encouraged for higher education in a family.
- Women who are responsible for feeding and educating their children are paid less for their labor than men.

The good news is that preventing maternal deaths is possible, even in resource-poor countries; but it requires the right kind of information. Recording numbers of deaths according to pregnancy-related definitions is not enough. We need to understand the underlying factors that lead to the deaths, which are pregnancy-*associated* causes of maternal mortality – and that includes poverty and low status of females in a masculine-valued society.

Identifying traditional biological threats to pregnant, childbearing, and postpartum women, intervening with pharmaceuticals or surgery, and associating a "cure" with seek-

and-destroy models based on scientific studies has helped to reduce some biological causes of disease and death. But perhaps we need to say what common sense, observation, and empirical evidence shows us: poverty and inaccessibility are the root causes of mothers' and newborns' deaths.

Sometimes, policy makers formulate health policy decisions based on "evidence" – so let's assure them that social and cultural risk factors are root causes for pregnancy-associated death. Applying new definitions for maternal mortality can be a step in the right direction. Decision-makers need to know that maternal and infant deaths can be avoided by raising the status of women in a society – by making sure that women count.

One way to do that is to assure competent care once a woman manages to arrive at the hospital. We all know how hospital staff are underpaid and overworked in every country and how the "brain-drain" of emigration from developing countries to the Northern or Western hemispheres causes staffing emergencies. So, you may ask, why don't we make use of all those traditional midwives in all those villages? She's the first line of defense anyway – the "go-to" person who does seem to have time for her clients. She exists in every village, in every urban barrio, in every suburb in *every* country. She has been present at all births since the beginning of time. Really, when you think about it, the traditional midwife may be the "oldest profession." So why hasn't she been trained to step up to the plate of interventionist medicine?

Because medicine is about authority and authority is about doctors. Let's look at one example of how integration of traditional midwives into the medical model of care involved the whole community – the traditional community and the medical community – and how that could have been a brilliant solution. Could have been.

Pregnant Pause

EVERY MINUTE OF EVERY DAY
SOMEWHERE ON PLANET EARTH:

360 women become pregnant.
190 of those are unplanned or unwanted.
110 pregnant women experience a
complication due to that pregnancy.
40 women have an unsafe abortion.

1 woman dies every minute from a pregnancy-related causes.

This woman may be 12 years old or 52 years old. She could be
your mother, your sister, your niece, or your wife. You could
be responsible for raising her other children. You could just
turn the page and give thanks you were not born a woman...

For more information and suggestions about
what you can do, wear a white ribbon and read all
about it: **www.thewhiteribbonalliance.org**

CHAPTER 4

Who are the Traditional Midwives?

The city of Sololá hovers in green hillsides, five hours by bus from Guatemala City. Blooming, blood-red bougainvilleas drape pastel-colored stucco walls. Donkeys loaded with fresh vegetables clip-clop down cobblestone streets from the surrounding mountain communities and bring fresh food to town. The Guatemalan traditional midwives – *comadronas* in Spanish – live in the mountainous villages around Sololá and bring most of their neighbors into the world. They say they became midwives by happenstance because they have attended so many births, or because they felt chosen by God. They see themselves, and others in their community see them, as the cultural authority on pregnancy, labor, birth, postpartum, and newborns.

Professional health providers in Sololá, graduates of medical and nursing schools, see themselves, and other professionals in the community see them, as the scientific authorities on pregnancy, labor, birth, postpartum, and newborns. The public hospital in Sololá sits between tall eucalyptus trees on a flat piece of land just above the hilly town. The hospital offers fifty beds, along with an operating room, with two "delivery" rooms. The administrator pulls nurses from other wards to attend a woman in labor because hospital births are such a rare event – whether that nurse is trained in obstetrics or not. In 1998, only 7% of babies in the entire province came into the world between elevated legs in cold steel stirrups on a gynecological table under bright lights inside the Sololá Hospital.

Guatemalan comadronas attend births at a woman's home the same way they have for centuries, with all the rituals and careful attention to details they learned from their mothers and grandmothers. Comadronas speak the same language as the mother (there are more than 150 native dialects in Guatemala). Comadronas spend more time with a mother at her home than a nurse can during a designated eight-hour shift at the hospital. Comadronas stay with the woman for days, nurture her with foods she likes to eat during labor and postpartum, give massages to alleviate labor pain, and perform precise rituals for the newborn that allow for a smooth transition from the spiritual world into its new earthly life.

In 1998, after fighting factions signed Peace Accords in Guatemala, government health personnel began to gather maternal and newborn health information – a project previously suspended for about 30 years due to the civil war. The public health doctors and nurses reviewed birth and death certificates and discovered that 90% of all births took place in the home with the comadrona. They interviewed women and comadronas and learned that pregnant woman avoided the hospital for many reasons – the least of which was the bad treatment they received.

The comadronas said hospital staff insulted their clients, yelled at them, and sometimes even slapped them. They said women preferred to avoid the humiliation. And besides, if a donkey ride down a hill during labor was the only form of transportation, most women preferred to labor in their own bed in their own home. The decision to seek medical care is made even more difficult by darkness. Taxi drivers, if you awakened one, sometimes charged a month's salary for their services to take you to the hospital.

A standoff existed between health professionals and the community: Women preferred the comadrona for her authority in their community; and the hospital staff blamed the comadrona for bringing in a woman too late to be saved if she had complications. Women and newborns continued to risk death by giving birth at home, and yet – as Sololá family physician Dr. Yadira de Cross discovered – many died on the way to, or inside the walls of, the Sololá hospital.

A short, petite woman with crinkle laugh-lines around her dark brown eyes, Yadira has an optimistic attitude that most of her colleagues call contagious. She took it upon herself to go out into the villages and meet with the community comadronas, to discover their level of expertise and why women chose their services instead of hers. What she heard was distressing and put a dent in her optimistic demeanor for days.

"Maternal death is not just *our* problem," she later explained to her colleagues one afternoon during the hospital's monthly Maternal Mortality Committee meeting. "It's a social problem. People are too poor to feed themselves, let alone find transportation to the hospital. Mothers trust the comadrona, even if she is illiterate and uneducated – and they don't trust us! When a mother dies in childbirth, the orphans are left to fend for themselves. The father and the entire family are devastated." She suggested forming local community health committees, or involving social workers to encourage more community participation in health issues that affect them.

It was past two o'clock in the afternoon, and no one on the hospital's Maternal Mortality Committee had eaten lunch yet. "Go ahead, Yadira, you do whatever you want," remarked a doctor, as he flipped the page to address the next issue on the agenda. "If you can find the funding," he added. When Yadira left at the end of the meeting, another woman followed her into the hallway.

Patricia de Leon Toledo, a Guatemalan sociologist completing her internship at the Sololá hospital, showed Yadira the data she'd collected from recent interviews of community members in the province. Her interviews showed that almost all births and maternal deaths occurred in the communities; deliveries in the hospital had worse outcomes than home births because patients arrived in the midst of an untreatable complication; people believed you only go to the hospital to die; no one liked the treatment in the hospital; husbands were the decision makers in the family, and most husbands in Sololá were out of the home for weeks at a time working in the coffee or banana plantations; the mothers-in-law seemed to be the secondary decision makers about whether or not to seek health care; and the community comadrona was seen as the principle authority for pregnancy, birth, postpartum, and newborn care. All of her data corroborated the Ministry of Health's surveys.

Yadira and Patricia then went online to review the Ministry of Health statistics for 2000 from January to June. Sololá had the highest estimated maternal and newborn mortality rates in all Guatemala – numbers that were probably underestimated due to poor birth and death registration in rural areas.

"I need some coffee," Yadira said with a sigh.

Patricia and Yadira later conferred with Ilse Santizo, an obstetrician from Guatemala City and specialist in public health. The three women decided to organize a district-wide meeting, the first of its kind in that part of Guatemala, to discover ways to decrease maternal and newborn death rates. They decided to involve everyone who had anything to do with women and babies in the province.

They invited obstetricians and nurses from the Sololá hospital and nearby private health centers to the meeting. They invited hospital management and local authorities from the communities, including evangelical pastors and schoolteachers. They invited the mayor of Sololá, the governor, Ministry of Health representatives from Guatemala City, the local news media, and the most popular daytime radio host in the province. They invited comadronas from twenty-three surrounding communities. They also invited mothers, their families, Catholic nuns, and the president of the taxi union – since taxi drivers were the ones who ended up taking a bleeding postpartum woman to the hospital at night. They called their forum *Primer Encuentro de Hablar Sobre la Mortalidad Materna en Sololá* – First Encounter to Talk about Maternal Mortality in Sololá.

Everyone crowded into the municipal meeting room near the main plaza during that hot August in 2000. TV news cameras with big floodlights covered the event, which added to the heat factor. Wooden floors and tables couldn't absorb the perspiration of 160 participants. High ceiling fans swirled stuffy air, and anticipation was humidity-thick. Dr. Yadira de Cross opened the forum by explaining, in layman's language, just exactly what is meant by the phrase "maternal mortality."

"If I told you '240 per 100,000 is the yearly maternal mortality ratio estimated for Guatemala,' you would probably start snoring," Yadira said to the fan-flapping crowd. "That is the way health statistics are measured. It means for every 100,000 babies born this year, 240 women will die. Any better?" she asked. She received blank stares and bobbing heads in reply.

"*Bueno*," she continued. "Let me put it another way. In Guatemala during this year, 970 women will die because they were pregnant or had a baby. That is the *total* number of dead women, not a ratio, according to estimates from the World Health Organization. These are numbers based on statistics given by our Ministry of Health. In other words, today, Monday, two or three women will die. On Tuesday also. On Wednesday, and every day, day after day, even on Sunday, all year long without stopping, two to three women will die from complications related to pregnancy or childbirth." She paused to let that fact sink in. Some mouths dropped open. No one spoke. Cameras panned the crowd.

"There will be no news stories," she said, paused, and looked right into the camera. "Nothing on the radio. No television reports about all these women dying. The only noise you'll hear will be the families crying over coffins before the burial."

People gasped and took notes. The mayor wanted answers. Health Ministry representatives exclaimed the evidence wasn't reliable. Doctors declared it wasn't their fault women didn't come to the hospital, where they could be saved. Comadronas said they didn't bring women to the hospital because they were sent away, forced to return to their villages without the mother – which to them was equal to "disappearing" their clients. Such fears echoed the kidnappings and killings that happened during the thirty-five-year Guatemalan civil war, when family members and whole villages were disappeared by government paramilitary forces and death squads. The Guatemalan Peace Accords had been signed only two years before.

"Why should we trust the government hospital now?" asked one comadrona.

"Blame" would have been the working word of the session, except that Patricia de Leon masterfully directed the discussions toward the four contributors to maternal and infant deaths. She called these causes "The Four Delays." The First Delay involves a lag in recognizing a danger sign, for example, hemorrhage or infection; the Second Delay concerns when/whether the decision-maker of the family chooses to seek help; the Third Delay entails finding available transportation to the hospital (everyone from the surrounding mountainous communities knew this one, and nodded in agreement); and the Fourth Delay involves receiving adequate and timely attention at the hospital or health post once you arrive. This last one ignited fiery debates between the hospital staff and the administrators about how, when, and which equipment or medicines are supplied to the hospital.

Patricia de Leon calmed the crowd and divided them into smaller working committees, assigning each group one of the Four Delays to discuss. Each group had to identify solutions for their assigned "Delay" – ways to improve health care and to decrease maternal mortality. The small groups would present their findings the next day.

On Tuesday, hospital personnel got an earful from men and women of the surrounding communities about the Second Delay – deciding to seek help.

"We know the comadrona can't do everything," said one new mother. "And we know where the hospital is. But we have many reasons for not coming down the mountain. We are Indians. The doctors are Ladinos (of Spanish descent). You know the rest." She sat down and crossed her brown arms over her chest, while her neighbors nodded their heads. The doctors looked straight ahead, their white hands under their chins.

Other women told how they hated the way they were treated when they came to the hospital, starting with the condescending attitude of the man at the door who decides whether or not to let them enter. Men stood up and said they hated it when they were kept outside, away from their wives, who need their protection.

More and more people, normally very shy about speaking in public, stood up to add to the list of complaints: They're not allowed to eat the foods they want at the hospital; they are humiliated in public; there is no privacy and strangers see their nakedness; they are degraded with pubic shaves and enemas; they hate having vaginal exams and IVs and cold rooms and no emotional support; the nurses even remove their newborns from their breasts! Many women who had never spoken to an authoritative figure like a doctor or governor before proclaimed their concerns in loud voices, and applauded when one woman said, "I would rather die in my home than go to that hospital and be humiliated."

The professional health providers addressed their assigned Fourth Delay: receiving adequate attention at the hospital once the woman arrived. They argued that the municipal and regional Ministry of Health authorities didn't provide them with adequate supplies, medications, or training.

"Our nurses on the night shift have no idea what to do when confronted with an obstetrical emergency," said one doctor. "How are we supposed to save a life if it takes me thirty minutes to get to the hospital at night and the nurse doesn't know what to do until I get there?"

As the Forum ground its way through the week, more and more information was shared, more and more fears were aired. Everyone agreed they wanted to prevent maternal and newborn deaths. They admitted they all needed to work together to accomplish the goals developed in their Action Plans that Friday afternoon. One of the Action Plans developed by the community members declared that each village must establish a local health committee that holds monthly meetings, and that they must report back to the district health official each month.

The community members defined in detail their health committee's responsibilities. For example, money would be collected for emergencies, thus making transport available. In San Pedro Sacatepéquez, each family must contribute one quetzal (equivalent to thirty US cents) every month to the "Emergency Health Fund." A pound of raw coffee beans from the nearby plantation cost about one quetzal, and most families could afford that amount. The money would be used to buy gasoline, pay a driver a small fee, and transport anybody in need of emergency care down the mountain to the hospital.

The regional representatives from the Ministry of Health also had an Action Plan. They promised to distribute necessary emergency obstetrical drugs and supplies to all government health facilities in Sololá province: oxytocin for prevention of postpartum hemorrhage, IV fluids for treating shock, and antibiotics for treating infections. They also promised to spend time and money on skills training for nurses to resolve obstetrical emergencies. They would even organize classes for the men who guarded the hospital emergency room door about how to be more "client friendly."

The doctors and nurses at Sololá hospital grudgingly came to recognize that comadronas could form an integral part of the formal health care system. They decided that their Action Plan would include a monthly meeting with the comadronas about how to make the hospital more acceptable to the woman and her family. Because of those monthly meetings, the labor ward now has curtains separating the beds for more privacy (sewn by the comadronas and sold to the hospital), nurses allow family members to be with the laboring woman, and mothers keep their newborns at their side.

After that first meeting many things changed. When a woman in the community had a problem or complication, the comadrona initiated the community's Emergency Response Network. The car, gasoline, driver, and family members responded to the call, and everyone accompanied the woman to the hospital. The comadrona and a family member stayed with the woman in the hospital during the resolution of the problem – whether cesarean or natural birth – and returned home with the mother and newborn, safe and sound.

Dedicated doctors, nurses, social workers, and community members put their concerns about mothers and newborns ahead of habits and fears. Dr. Estuardo Flores, at that time a director at the Guatemala Ministry of Health, said, "We have proven that comadronas are a very useful connection between the hospital and the community."

Unfortunately, this story does not end "Happily Ever After." Allowing comadronas to accompany women into the Sololá hospital didn't even last two years. No one trained the comadronas in how to intervene in their isolated villages if they recognized a danger sign. The government physicians didn't *want* a comadrona intervening. And government-trained nurses at the hospital continued to train the comadronas about the importance of *transfer* – as in, get her down the mountain and into the hospital, where we professionals can treat her! Those same professionals insist that they alone are the authority in their community of practice. They don't *want* to train traditional midwives to step in and redefine their role, replace the nurses' responsibility, or occupy their ownership as The Authority on health.

Government training programs for the village midwife always result in maintaining a status quo defined by the government health policy – and more importantly, sustains in place those whom the *government* (not the people) trusts as the health authority in the villages. What most non-governmental people recognize is that intervention for illness needs to be dealt with on a spiritual/ emotional level, and not only the physical. People who have not been inundated with promises from the pharmaceutical industry believe that imbalance causes illness, and bringing someone back to balance involves much more than medication and surgery.

Thus we may understand the important role of the traditional midwife, and not only in Guatemala or even Latin America. Traditional healers in every culture, throughout the ages, have always emphasized the importance of a spiritual and emotional balance of one's place in the bigger scheme of things, with good physical health that naturally follows the balance. Our educational systems for nurses and doctors, unfortunately, deflate or diminish the importance of these other concepts that cannot be "measured" scientifically, to our personal and social detriment.

Let's see an example of how difficult it is to change behaviors and habits based on what we know and trust to be "true" – which is based on an erroneous educational system.

Pregnant Pause

A group of European midwives founded the International Confederation of Midwives (ICM) in 1919 in Belgium.

ICM Definition of a Midwife

A midwife is a person who, having been regularly admitted to a midwifery educational program duly recognized in the country in which it is located, has successfully completed the prescribed course of studies in midwifery and has acquired the requisite qualifications to be registered and/or legally licensed to practice midwifery.

The midwife is recognized as a responsible and accountable professional who works in partnership with women to give the necessary support, care, and advice during pregnancy, labour, and the postpartum period, to conduct births on the midwife's own responsibility and to provide care for the newborn and the infant. This care includes preventive measures, the promotion of normal birth, the detection of complications in mother and child, the accessing of medical or other appropriate assistance, and the carrying out of emergency measures.

The midwife has an important task in health counseling and education, not only for the woman, but also within the family and community. This work should involve antenatal education and preparation for parenthood, and may extend to women's health, sexual or reproductive health, and childcare.

A midwife may practice in any setting including in the home, the community, hospitals, clinics, or health units.

In 1982, Canadian, Mexican, and US midwives organized the Midwives Alliance of North America (MANA).

MANA Statement of Values

WE VALUE

- Women and their creative, life-affirming, and life-giving powers, which find expression in a diversity of ways.
- The oneness of the pregnant mother and her unborn child – an inseparable and interdependent whole.
- The integrity of life's experiences – the physical, emotional, mental, psychological, and spiritual components of a process are inseparable.
- Pregnancy and birth as natural processes that technology will never supplant.
- Pregnancy and birth as personal, intimate, internal, sexual, and social events to be shared in the environment and with the attendants a woman chooses.
- A mother's intuitive knowledge of herself and her baby before, during, and after birth.
- A woman's innate ability to nurture her pregnancy and birth her baby – the power and beauty of her body as it grows and the awesome strength summoned in labor.
- The essential mystery of birth.
- Our relationship to a process larger than ourselves, recognizing that birth is something we can seek to learn from and know, but never control.
- Expertise that incorporates academic knowledge, clinical skill, intuitive judgment, and spiritual awareness.
- Relationship – the quality, integrity, equality, and uniqueness of our interactions inform and critique our choices and decisions.

CHAPTER 5

How is Society Threatened?

People in the United States accustomed to private illness care driven by economic factors (excluding those accustomed to socialized medicine in the form of US Armed Services health care, the Bureau of Indian Affairs, or Medicaid/Medicare) may not understand that public health in most countries is physician-directed, capital city-located, public-funds salaried, and political-party appointed -- all of which dictate what happens at each public health institution, from health post to hospital. And when governing political parties change, political appointments change on almost every level.

Doctors have only their political connections and forceful personalities to promote themselves within a public health system that pays a pittance. From Algeria to Zimbabwe, the "lowly" general practitioner may get that longed-for recommendation to attend specialty training in the capital, or the hospital director may have a better chance at becoming a university professor – a position that imitates bankers' hours from Monday to Friday: no nights or weekends or holidays – *if* they go along with whatever their brother physicians at the Ministry of Health deem to be Correct Medical Practice. Even better, avoiding ruffling fellow-physician feathers may lead toward a position within the Ministry of Health!

Also, you never know who is going to be your boss after the next change of government. That colleague you confronted in the delivery room by promoting the presence of comadronas in the hospital may be giving you marching orders the very next year if he is assigned to be the Chief of Staff by the new incoming government's Minister of Health. "If you like the comadronas so much, why don't we just assign you to the Health Post out there in the mountains for a couple of years? You can work with hemorrhages and infections, with no back-up, as much as you like!"

The obstetricians in Sololá never really accepted idea of working with comadronas. Why should they accept competition within their territory? After all, they believed traditional midwives were the cause of most maternal death and disease. If pregnant women would come to the hospital in the first place, doctors declared, we wouldn't have all these problems!

Cornelia Muhl, a German midwife charged with training comadronas by her employer, Midwives for Midwives (a Guatemala non-governmental organization),[25] did bring comadronas into the Sololá hospital – after exhaustive personal meetings with the doctor at the Ministry of Health in charge of Reproductive Health for the country. That doctor (recently appointed to his post because of a change in government) ended up *ordering* the obstetricians at Sololá to accept a temporary truce and, for the sake of scientific study, to accept some traditional midwives for practical skills training at the hospital...for two months.

Hired from Hamburg by Midwives for Midwives in Guatemala, graduated from a five-year university midwifery program with five years of hospital practice, and loaded with good Spanish language skills along with good intentions, Cornelia arrived in January from freezing Germany to tropical Guatemala. From February to April of 2005, she worked alongside 28 comadronas and four rural nurses in the Sololá hospital, nights, weekends, holidays, and any other time a laboring woman needed a midwife at her side for prenatal care, childbirth, postpartum, newborn attention, or family planning counseling. Cornelia used a training package with checklists and learning guides developed specifically for less-literate comadronas, so she could objectively teach and measure the midwives' skills. These skills included measuring blood pressure, taking a woman's vital signs, checking the position of the fetus with special hands-on maneuvers, timing the contractions, learning when a labor is prolonged and what to do if it is, massaging for pain reduction, resuscitating the adult and newborn, learning the importance of breastfeeding immediately after birth, practicing normal newborn care, and preventing postpartum hemorrhage, among other abilities. It is important to note that *none* of these skills had ever been taught to comadronas in Guatemala before – the very people who attend 90% of all births.

Remember, nurses from the Ministry of Health government training programs are instructed to teach traditional midwives how to mind their own business and not replace the professionals, and to do only two things well: recognize danger signs and transfer. The nurses emphasize that "only professionally trained doctors and nurses" should care for a woman during her pregnancy and birth. This is not just a phenomenon of Guatemala or even Latin America, but worldwide.

Cornelia, the German midwife, wrote in her final report for Midwives For Midwives that, "At first, the hospital personnel thought I must be a doctor training the midwives, even though I explained my degree and professional midwifery status. They couldn't imagine a midwife as a professional. I guess believing I was a physician made them feel better about my presence." She also objectively and professionally noted which skills the comadronas and nurses learned well, and which ones they had difficulty with. She reported on the eleven-week training results with German precision:

- We had ten clinical days for each student, consisting of 7-8 hours a day, plus some overnight shifts of 12 hours, and some overtime when we had births. The average was 80 to 90 hours of clinical training per student.
- Each student had an average of three births: two as assistant and one as the principal midwife.
- Students attended 32 births, 4 of which were C-sections for failure to progress, defined by the doctor on duty.
- Students resuscitated (successfully) three babies. No babies died from our attendance.

- Students had one perineal tear (second degree), and students only had to cut one episiotomy.
- Of 111 prenatal appointments, each student had an average of five clients.
- Each student learned to do a complete clinical history and prenatal physical assessment, i.e., fundal heights measurements, fetal heart counting and listening, fetal position and presentation, vital signs, and counseling.
- Students gave postnatal care to 192 postpartum women, an average of 8 to 14 each.

It bears repeating that none of these skills or competencies had *ever* been taught to the traditional midwives before in any government-sponsored class. The midwives' tears of gratitude dampened their certificates during their graduation ceremony.

Cornelia rarely showed emotion in her final report for Midwives for Midwives. In one instance she mentions that the students were very good about using the checklists, and they "...were very self-confident after the first month, and proud of themselves for the good job they did."

Only once did Cornelia offer an emotive and diplomatic insight about staff relationships. She wrote, "As we all know, to start working in the hospital was very hard. We encountered hostility with nurses and doctors every day. With time we started to make friends, and they started seeing us as helpers for their work. They did not give many prenatal appointments to us, but by the end they were giving us almost all their patients. With time we demonstrated that we were safe caregivers. They saw that we could resuscitate babies, that we were able to conduct births safely and with intact perineums, that we could repair tears, that we could examine babies and help women to be safe and with good care. By the end they all knew that we used music, we allowed family to be with women, and that we used different positions for giving birth. In the last week they gave us two laboring women a day, maybe because they knew we were leaving."

Cornelia and the other professional midwives working with Jenna Houston, founder and director of Midwives for Midwives, had much more to say personally about the treatment they and the mothers received in the hospital. They are horror stories, really, about doctors cursing comadronas in front of their clients, about professionals preferring the finals of the regional soccer playoff on TV to the six women they had in labor, about losing blood samples, misplacing medications, or not charting untoward events from their erroneous interventions, thus preventing subsequent investigation.

These practices are not rare or even unusual. But it's also not hard to understand why doctors and nurses are territorial about their hospital rituals and practice (see Chapter 9). Their training, fears, and habits guide them to want to control the outcome.

While childbirth is pretty unpredictable, it doesn't have to be panicky. But to follow the ebbs and tides of birthing, to know when the woman needs guidance to get back into the flow if she's floundering, demands attendance, observation, caring, and concern. That takes time. If one nurse has four or fifteen patients, she has no time to spend with any of them. One doctor on call for an entire village or hospital needs to sleep, too.

The Midwives Association of North America (MANA), the International Association of Midwives (IAM), and other organizations[26] recognize and respect traditional midwifery practices (recognizing that education and training is necessary during all our careers – be that traditional midwifery or university-graduated midwifery). They understand that women who value women for their creative powers are no threat to society: *They are the reason that society survives.* One of the most significant statements in the MANA list of Midwifery Values[27] is the following:

> We value our relationship to a process larger than
> ourselves, recognizing that birth is something we can
> seek to learn from and know, but never control.

Midwives – and physicians who promote the midwifery model – recognize that the medicalization of childbirth generates more problems than it solves. Health care becomes illness care, because that's where the economic reimbursement comes from. When physicians are "gatekeepers" of information or of the legalization of careers, patients have restricted choice of alternative or non-invasive medical procedures and out-of hospital care. As we all know, medicalization is very costly in private systems like the U.S., and for societies in general like those systems in Canada or the European Union. The medicalization of "health" care is bound to encourage medical interventions for the highest financial return, rather than cheaper options that often produce better outcomes for patients.[28] High C-section rates are just one example.

Statistics support the midwifery model of care. Just look at any year since records were kept (from the mid-1800s) in both Europe and the Nordic countries: records prove the comparatively low perinatal mortality rates (pregnancy, childbirth, and postpartum) and infant mortality rates wherever midwives are the primary caregivers. Of course, these statistics involve educated girls and women, higher rates of economic income, better nutrition, excellent access to services, and contraceptive care – all the sociological factors mentioned that impact mother or child death rates.

One of the great controversies dividing pregnant women, midwives, physicians, and Ministries of Health officials over the past ten years remains: Do we train traditional midwives in life-saving skills, or not? Many studies have been done about this subject and others: Do we train more professionals and upgrade the hospital infrastructure? Why can't we do both? Who has the money for all this? What do we consider to be "measurable outcomes" for all this intervention? Do we have the time to wait for midwifery students to graduate from a four-year course and get out into the rural areas to see any results? Is she even accepted in rural areas by the people she serves? Most studies over the past ten years have shown that professional providers (midwives or doctors or nurses) *may* be accepted by the rural folk if and when they see immediate results that are beneficial to their physical health. But when it comes to spiritual and emotional health, the village midwife remains the best hedge against unforeseen circumstances, despite her lack of training.

Of course, government Ministries of Health in poorer countries don't agree. In a study from the University of Nairobi in Kenya, the authors conclude that, "Despite tremendous resources spent on them, the training of Traditional Birth Attendants* over the

---

* Traditional Birth Attendants are otherwise known as "TBAs," a deprecatory title used by most university-educated professionals for traditional midwives. These women call themselves midwives.

past two decades...has not reduced maternal mortality."[29] They credit any observed improvement after introducing TBA training programs (*government-dictated* programs, given by university-educated nurses) to the associated "supervision and referral systems," or to the quality of essential obstetric services available at first referral level. First level means the health post. It could also mean the home, if the midwife was adequately trained in life-saving skills, or if the mother, the midwife, or the nurse had access to adequate supplies at the first-level referral center.

This study (and many similar ones) mentions that a family's continued preference for traditional midwives is attributed to proximity to the woman's home, respectful attitude toward the mother and her family, and flexible modes of payment – things apparently lacking at the government health center. The Kenya study also points out that "distance and access to skilled attendance are factors that influence maternal deaths rates." How can the "TBA" resolve that *government's* problem? And how can any government "dismiss" the traditional midwife?

According to a respected South African literary magazine,[30] "Traditional midwives have been an integral part of African medicine for centuries. This is not only because African people still love and fear the spirits, but also because a great number of the South African population do not have access to existing health services."

If you search the Google web site for "traditional midwife" you will find more than 861,000 entries. Much as they are ignored, deprecated, illegalized, or trained to be something they are not, traditional midwives have always existed, since the beginning of time...the world's oldest profession.

Meanwhile, in Kenya, Guatemala, Indonesia, China, Paraguay, even the USA – wherever traditional midwives continue to serve women's and families' physical, spiritual, and emotional needs in their communities – government doctors in charge of health policy for populations will continue to try to convince folks that they need to trust the institution of medicine and all its technology. Curing and rescue interventions are quicker and easier than building health facilities, building roads to reach them, equipping them, staffing them, training and paying staff, educating girls, or eradicating poverty.

Training traditional midwives to just "recognize danger signs and transfer" will not save more lives, because that philosophy disconnects the family, the decision-makers in the community, and the spiritual, emotional, or psychological components of pregnancy and childbirth. When governments begin to connect all these dots, maybe the resulting paint-by-number image will show us the Big Picture of health care. Perhaps when giving life matters more than taking life, our priorities will point the way toward eradicating poverty: resulting in better nutrition, better hygiene, less malaria, STD and HIV, and better access to safe interventions at low cost. When giving life matters more than taking life, and when the person giving life matters more than the person taking life (soldiers), then health care, not illness care, will become national priorities. And what better model to show the way than the midwifery model? – a model like the one offered by the Midwives Alliance of North America, which declares midwives "value expertise, which incorporates academic knowledge, clinical skill, intuitive judgment, and spiritual awareness."

One way to incorporate traditional and other midwives into a medical model is to allow midwives to bring their clients into the hospital and stay with them. Then, the patient gets the best of both worlds: the midwifery model based on trust that birth works, and the medical model of care based on intervention in case of emergency.

Chile has a very good medical model to study – and avoid – that demonstrates the interventionist, separatist, medical model of care that has supplanted the long and healthy history of midwifery care in that country. This medical model, designed and deemed preferable by physicians, confers upon Chile the highest government-financed cesarean-section surgery rate in the world. Let's see how Chile eradicated their traditional midwives slowly and surely, and how most of the university-trained mini-medicos who call themselves *matronas* (Chilean Spanish for midwives) maintain and encourage obstetrician-directed interventions.

Pregnant Pause

There is a distinction between the bio-technical and "modern" model of health care, compared with the humanistic, or holistic, model of health care that we see everywhere around us. The distinction is especially evident between medical care and traditional midwifery care for the pregnant and birthing woman and her newborn.

TECHNOCRATIC MODEL OF CARE
BASIC PRINCIPLE = *SEPARATION*

1. Mechanization of the body
2. Isolation and the objectification of the patient
3. Focus on curing disease, repairing dysfunction
4. Aggressive, interventionist approach to diagnosis and treatment
5. Alienation of practitioner from patient
6. Reliance on external diagnosis
7. Super valuation of technology
8. Hierarchical organization (patient is subordinate to practitioner and to institution)
9. Authority and responsibility inherent in the practitioner

HUMANISTIC MODEL OF CARE:
BASIC PRINCIPLE = *RESPECT*

1. The individual is to be valued as unique and worthy.
2. The body is an organism, not a machine.
3. The whole person should always be considered.
4. The needs of the individual and the institution should be balanced.

5. Information, decision-making, and responsibility should be shared between provider and patient.
6. Empathetic communication – including eye contact and touch – is essential to healing.

These two models of care were developed and published by anthropologist Robbie Davis-Floyd, Ph.D., and presented at the International Conference on Humanization of Childbirth in Fortaleza, Brazil, in November 2000.

CHAPTER 6

Is Health Policy Economic Policy?

In most Latin American societies, sameness and conformity are much more comfortable, valued, and promoted than are British or North American traits like individuality or non-conformity. Obeying the rules brings social acceptance (very important to class-conscious people with rigid mores), while individuality breeds anarchy and possible revolution (anyone with a different viewpoint could be labeled a "Communist" and shunned, shot, or disappeared). Jorge Castaneda said in a *Newsweek* editorial (Feb 22, 1999), "We Latin Americans are likely to fear any threat to the status-quo and oppose after-the-fact investigations." Thus we see the benign acceptance of a culture of corruption in Mexico, of an endless cycle of poverty and NGO handouts in Bolivia and Ecuador, of street killings in Brazil, of torture and genocide in the Central American highlands, of 75% C-section rates by doctors in private hospitals with no oversight except by other doctors, and of total white, middle-class standardization in Chile, Uruguay, and Argentina.

Other Latin American countries look upon these last three countries, especially Chile, as a role model for their medical systems. According a Peruvian doctor I met: "The reason we all want to imitate the Chilean system is because it works so well for the medical community. And the reason it works so well is because Chile doesn't have an Indian problem."

Before the Spaniards came, of course, original peoples existed in every country in the Western Hemisphere. In southern Chile their name is Mapuche. Hundreds of thousands of indigenous populations existed before smallpox, venereal disease, rape, murder, and guns exterminated the majority of them. The Mapuche have the honor of being the only native people in Chile to never have been conquered by the Spaniards.

Naturally, original peoples had their own health system, like all indigenous peoples everywhere, with their own cosmology, based on empirical (not scientific) evidence. Pablo Manquenahuel, a Mapuche poet, writes, "We do not separate the universe from nature, or humans from society. We do not feel we are the owners of nature because we are part of Her. If anything, we are Her children and She cares for us. Because of these beliefs, there is no superior or inferior, only diversity. Difference is the wonder of life."[31]

This sounds suspiciously pagan these days, but illuminates a way of viewing the world and our place in it that can still be found on every continent, in every country, in every culture that connects spiritual health with physical health, and connects the seen with the unseen. Dividing things down to the most microscopic degree in order to understand, conquer, and control them is very Greek and military. Yet while this process helps define causes of diseases, it becomes deadly when determining health care. (We'll see more of the history of the medical focus on health in Chapter 12.)

My uncle was a professor of military ethics and head of the Department of Philosophy at Texas A&M University until he retired. He reminded me that good, fertile ground for sprouting any authoritarian government arises when citizens prefer security to liberty. Authoritarian figures always give us the illusion of comfort and of security, which may be why 98% of Chilean pregnant women want a (hopefully male) doctor to attend their births instead of a perfectly competent matrona (Chilean midwife); why women request and receive ultrasound exams for *every* prenatal visit; and why there is a 75% rate of cesarean operations in public hospitals and up to 95% in private hospitals![32]

A culture inherited from the Spanish conquistadors and blended with the rigid mores of the Catholic Church, which insists upon and rewards recognition of vertical authoritarian systems, dominates and defines Chile's value system. For example, the "patron" is the person who pays your salary, guarantees you a place to live, subsidizes your kids' education, and arranges social events for the "peons." The priest is your intermediary with God, and through rituals of baptism, blessings, and burial ceremonies, assures you a good seat on the bus to the afterlife. The police along with the military are the ultimate authority figures for a "functioning" society, and the doctor and his representatives, including university-trained midwives, are the authority figures with control over birth and death – the operative word here being "control" with its "reassuring appearance of sameness and conformity to the socially dominant reality model."[33]

Anthropologist Brigitte Jordan pointed to this model of authority and conformity when she wrote, "In hospital deliveries, responsibility and credit are clearly the physician's. This becomes visible in the handshake and 'thank-you' that resident and intern (or intern and medical student) exchange after birth. 'Good work' is a compliment to a physician by somebody qualified to judge, namely another physician. Typically, nobody thanks the woman. In the common view, she has *been delivered* rather than given birth."[34]

The National System of Health Services governs health care in Chile. This universal health care system, developed in 1952 by then-Minister of Health Dr. Salvador Allende, was formally restructured in 1983 during the military government of Augusto Pinochet and became implemented by Pinochet's appointed ministers when the military junta began imposing private reforms in the economic realm. The idea was to rescue those sectors such as mining, manufacturing, military, and agriculture by redistributing funds from education and health to those with more earning potential.

While Minister of Health, Dr. Allende sponsored a law mandating 3.8% of Chile's gross national product to go toward universal health care for all citizens. After getting rid of Allende, Pinochet and his conservative cronies rearranged the health budget, which bombed to 0.8% of the GNP for two decades and has only managed to crawl back up to 3% under Dr. Michelle Bachelet's democratically elected socialist government since 2004.[35]

In 1954 the Chilean government began a campaign to get rid of all their traditional midwives. Chile has had university-trained midwives, or matronas, since 1834, trained by physicians and using medical textbooks from then until today, under the auspices of a university's School of Medicine. Matronas then and now are legally permitted to attend births at home, in a clinic, or in a hospital; but how they receive compensation for this care has been relegated to the fine print of their legal standing.

During the 1950s, while doctors still made private house calls (mostly for the rich), traditional midwives were encouraged to see their patients within the public health clinic setting and began to be paid a salary *by the state* (not their clients). The government's propaganda machine in the press and radio encouraged women to not pay the traditional midwife directly – the government would pay her a salary. The government then encouraged traditional midwives to bring their clients to the professional midwives for prenatal care, and paid the traditional midwife a small head-fee for this client capture. Remember, conformity was then and continues to be a very powerful social motivator in Chile. If my neighbor goes to the university-trained midwife, then I will also. If my health ministry tells me it's better for me to go to a professional, then I trust that authority.

The Ministry of Health (directed by physicians, don't forget) ensured in the early years that the federal government would subsidize only prenatal and postnatal visits by midwives, however, not hospital visits. The reimbursement plan insisted upon the separation between prenatal and labor/delivery care, the latter of which must happen in a hospital. The governmental system then paid a *separate* midwife (university trained) to attend births in the hospital. Only the physician, also reimbursed by the state, could see the client during her prenatal visits *and* her labor and childbirth *and* her postpartum visits. Thus, only the physician remained a constant presence in a pregnant woman's care, assuring the connection of the woman to her doctor, and disconnecting her from her midwife.

Separation of midwifery staff, along with the promotion of one doctor-one patient, became the hallmark of the Chilean model of health care, including payment reimbursement by the government to the hospital or health center, not by the client to the health provider. Who would you trust for your health care? Someone you saw for every visit and knew would be with your during the birth of your baby? Or someone you knew you would never see again? The medical profession slowly and surely took over the midwifery profession – and continues to this day.

Traditional midwives could not compete in that economic structure, and according to the cultural value for conservative conformity, women went along with what was dictated: the Doctor Knows Best. It took almost 25 years, but eventually the older, traditional midwives died out and the young, energetic ones took over – under the supervision of physicians from the Ministry of Health, of course.

At the end of the day, Chilean women trust absolutely in an authoritative personality outside themselves, and not in their own internal authoritative process about pregnancy and birth. Matronas are trained to promote this outside authority, and the legislature happily follows instructions from the doctors. In Chile's current public health care finance scheme, federal laws dictate that a flat reimbursement fee from the Ministry of Health goes to the health center via the municipality where a woman receives her prenatal care. This reimbursement fee is based on client count; thus, the more patients seen per hour, the more the municipality pipes money into your public health center, which pays your salary. If you live in a small community with only a few hundred pregnant women, then your health center does not receive many funds. Any obstetrician working for a public health center is allowed and encouraged to have their private practice on the side to supplement their income. This model for public health medicine can be found in almost every country.

The federal government reimburses hospitals directly without going through the municipality, and also compensates per client count. Interestingly, the more clients you care for in a twelve-hour period, the more the government pays your hospital. Even more interesting, the government pays *exactly the same rate* for a vaginal birth as for a scheduled C-section. Now, why would a doctor or hospital administrator who receives that kind of reimbursement wait for one woman to labor for twelve hours, when five women could receive Cesareans in that same amount of time?

It may help to recall that in the United States, way back in 1905, an editorial in the *Journal of the American Medical Association* declared that their profession was "at the starving point" from having admitted so many women into medical schools in the late 1890s. The feminization of the profession had resulted in an inevitable decrease in salary and prestige. The American Medical Association affirmed that the standing and influence of the profession depended on "the material success and financial independence of its members."[36] That policy pervades every medical society.

The medical approach to childbirth and women's health, throughout the world and not only in Chile, resembles an economic managerial process concerned with organizing time/money issues, along with preventing the inevitable mechanical breakdown of the human machine. Managed care, as it is sometimes referred to, really means "control over," and not "flowing with." It calls for conquering nature to avoid disaster, instead of working with nature to rejoice in her wisdom. In Chile, and in other countries where physicians make laws about our bodies, separation is highly valued, while connection is feared.

Jeanne Achterberg, in her powerful work *Woman As Healer,*[37] reminds us that honoring life is the real essence of the healing arts, be that medicine, midwifery, nursing, or any other healing art. All other discussions are trivial in comparison. Honoring life is also about honoring death, which also honors the exquisite richness of existence. She emphasizes that the call to honor life is not a value statement about "abortion rights," but rather a "warning of the devastation that occurs when women's individual responsibility is lost. When governments and other social institutions determine reproductive control, then abortions, birth control, pro-natal policy, or infanticide are just as likely to be mandated."[38] And when societies dictate life as surplus, it is usually the girl babies who are aborted, sold, or exposed. I agree with Acterberg's statement that "the greatest mischief in medicine has occurred because life was not honored." We who have worked in public health systems around the world have seen firsthand the doctor's ego preferred over the life of a woman or infant. It's the classic, common, and tragic scene where the doctor says, "I've got an important meeting. Let's get that baby out!"

From the extreme example of the medical model gone mad, we may also glimpse what happens to a society that values a medical/masculine system more than women's own internal authority. The maternal and infant death rate is low in Chile, compared to other Latin American countries, but that is not due to medical intervention; it's due to good nutrition, contraception, and public health systems.

Remember how counting maternal deaths depends upon who does the defining? The number one cause of women's death, and *not counted as maternal mortality* in Chile, is abortion – in a country that defines all abortion as illegal.

Let's look at another country with a medical interventionist system of care that tries desperately to lower their maternal mortality rate – a rate whose numbers are defined as "death by hemorrhage."

Pregnant Pause

Only around 15% of women ever develop a complication during their pregnancy, or birth or postpartum period. But nobody knows who belongs to that pesky 15%.

There is no such thing as a "high risk" pregnancy!

Any woman who is pregnant runs the risk (a small one, but still there) of developing a life-threatening complication. So it's better to *plan your pregnancy* (wanted and well-nourished), *space* your pregnancies (two to three years between gestations), or *not get pregnant.* Remember: A well-nourished, loving pregnancy means a very high chance of having a Happy Birth Day and a life long love affair with your baby and your Self.

CHAPTER 7

Is Prevention Cost Effective?

More than 200 million people live on the 17,508 islands that constitute the largest archipelago state in the world, home to the world's largest Muslim population. Inhabited originally by "Java Man" about 2 million years ago, their descendants took advantage of the fertile fields and warm climates to live and prosper on what later became known as the "Spice Islands." The name Indonesia, derived from the Greek *Indus*, meaning "India" and *nesos*, meaning "islands," describes the fourth most populated country in the world, dispersed over a land mass of six longitudes, two latitudes, two times zones, two oceans, and two hemispheres.

This is not a geography lesson...but just take a minute to look at the map below. Can't you just imagine romantic beaches on many of those 17,000 islands? Or the swaying palms, and the most diverse flora and fauna on the planet? Fresh fruit, rolling hills covered in tea plantations, abundance from the sea – a paradise. For our public health purposes, however, I tend to look at a map for cities that may have a referral hospital.

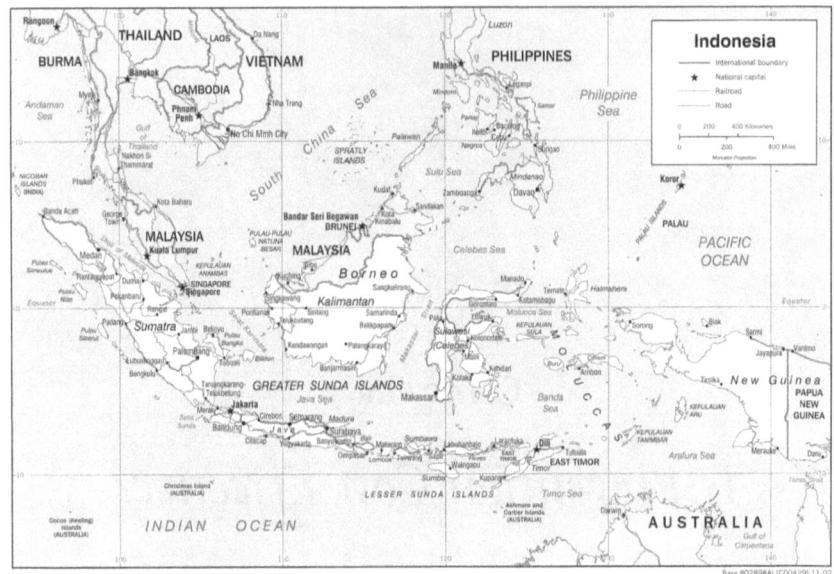

The main Indonesian island, Java, with its contaminated capital of Jakarta, has quite a few hospitals. Southern Borneo has a couple. Aceh may have one or two hospitals left after the devastating 2004 tsunami devoured everything – but with the guerrilla war still going on, it may be difficult to get to a hospital there, especially at night. The same goes for Guinea. Each of the remaining *thousands* of islands may have a small government health center staffed by dedicated nurses, midwives, or doctors working there on their obligatory year of provincial service to pay back their student loans. Or they may not. If not, a pregnant woman bleeding from a miscarriage may have to die at home – if she has a home.

According to the 2006 CIA "World Fact Book,"[39] the number of internally homeless persons in Aceh alone hovers around 570,000, with nearly 500,000 on the other big island provinces of Kalimantan, Maluku, New Guinea, and Central Sulawesi. Having a home or health care, in other words, is dicey in paradise.

Fortunately, we have the *bidan de desa*, the village midwife. This representative of the world's oldest profession (who attended Java Man's mother during his birth) can be found in every village, on every island. Of course, like other traditional midwives, she may or may not have received sanctioned training from the government du jour. She may or may not be educated enough in emergencies. But she is *there*. And what's more important, the people of her community believe in her and go to her for their spiritual, emotional, and physical health care. They may or may not decide to go see the doctor or the university-educated midwife at the rural health post, dutifully sitting watch during their year-long assignment from the Ministry of Health. After all, they have just recently graduated from school, they do not belong to any family in the village, and they act like they are above the rest of the people. This is not only a problem in Indonesia, but in all areas where doctors are not "on call" except for the very wealthy or in the capital cities where the very wealthy live. In one Indonesian health care study,[40] the main factor contributing to maternal death (77%) was the delay in decision making – to decide whether to go to the health center or not. The next greatest factor for maternal mortality in that study (60%) was the poor quality of care at the facility once the laboring woman arrived.

Doctors in Indonesia, and everywhere else, believe that *distance from their interventions = disaster-deliveries*, and they proceed to tweak public policy in an attempt to deliver health care for the most people with the least resources. And in Indonesia, that covers many people over *many* islands. One of their tweakings involved training the village bidan de desa.

From 1994 to 1998, the US non-governmental organization MotherCare sent professional Certified Nurse Midwives to the big island of Kalimantan – home of the Kalimantan Gold Corporation, which boasts exploration rights over the "largest and lowest cost copper-gold deposits in the world."[41] The government of Indonesia asked the US midwives to train the university-educated Indonesian midwives, along with the village bidan de desas in the remote mountain and jungle areas, to learn lifesaving skills and to demonstrate the Indonesian government's concern toward their non-foreign, gold-digging constituents.

MotherCare did a good job and had many success stories during their five-year tenure.[42] One important and simple preventive measure taught by midwives to midwives involved interpersonal communication skills training, for example, to explain what anemia is and why it's important to prevent anemia during pregnancy. In the MotherCare intervention, the likelihood of a pregnant woman receiving information about taking iron pills (which helps prevent anemia) went from 0 to 83%, and that woman's chances of understanding what anemia is and how it may lead to hemorrhage went from 6 to 73%![43] At the end of the successful five-year training program by midwives for midwives, however, their financial sponsor, USAID (United States Agency for International Development, a branch within the US Department of State), removed the funding for this prevention program and redirected the next five-year, multi-million-dollar project toward one that trains doctors and university midwives in emergency obstetric interventions in hospital settings, to treat hemorrhage (resulting from anemia).

If a woman does manage to make it to a hospital, she should then receive the best care possible to stop the bleeding, to cure an infection, to surgically deliver a stuck baby, or to stop eclampsia convulsions (the five top causes of death for mothers in Indonesia) – that is, if she manages to make it to the hospital....

We have to remember, also, that on average only 10-15% of all births result in emergencies that need intervention; and while 85-90% of all pregnant women are anemic not all of them will hemorrhage. Also, 85-90% of all births are normal events and Happy Birth Days. The trick is to guess which one will be the disaster delivery.

Programs to *prevent* hemorrhage, eclampsia, infection, or obstructed labor remain at the bottom of funding agencies' agendas because interventions come under a doctor's control; interventions involve diagnosis, treatment and hospitals; and, these interventions are easier to investigate and publish in "randomized, controlled, double blind" studies. Public health programs that emphasize prevention (like anti-tetanus vaccinations, anti-malaria bed-nets, and iron pills to prevent anemia) are nice but, let's face it, pharmaceutical companies and other big spenders are not interested – even though the prevention programs, like those of MotherCare, have been proven to work! Developing countries' Ministries of Health want the big bucks from big donors to do the big investigations and interventions; they need the money to pay their salaries and survive in their jobs, after all.

Thus, the Indonesia Ministry of Health and the Johns Hopkins School of Public Health (with USAID money) funded a study[44] to find a way stem the flow of women bleeding to death during immediate postpartum involving intervention instead of prevention. Prevention of hemorrhage, in Indonesia's case, could have focused on malaria eradication, nutritional subsidies for poor populations, and free iron pills for pregnant women – all precursors to anemia which may lead to hemorrhage in childbirth

However, Indonesian doctors wanted a pharmaceutical intervention. They found one in several small white pills called misoprostol – an ulcer medication – that when taken by the new mother immediately after the birth of her placenta slows down and may even halt bleeding! Many other studies[45] just like the one in Indonesia were conducted in several countries using rigorous international scientific standards involving university doctoral candidates, epidemiologists, professors, statisticians, Ministry of Health physicians and, oh yes, pregnant women.

Here's how it works (and it works quite well): a woman takes two pills immediately after she expels her placenta. The active ingredient in the anti-ulcer pills, prostaglandin, helps the uterus to contract, thus preventing hemorrhage from a "boggy" uterus. She takes two more pills four hours later. Of course, all these studies recommend a skilled attendant at birth who knows what to do for the *other causes of hemorrhage* besides a non-contracted uterus – an attendant who knows how to sew a torn cervix or perineum, for example, or repair a ruptured uterus, or who can manually remove a stuck placenta. These unpredictable but not uncommon problems also cause deadly postpartum hemorrhage, and the anti-ulcer drug misoprostol (whose main ingredient is prostaglandin) has no effect on any of these other causes of hemorrhage.

But we'll try the misoprostol. During a woman's prenatal visit, the skilled attendant (university trained midwife or nurse or doctor) gives the pregnant woman four misoprostol pills and explains when to take them, what to look for in case they don't work, and what to do if bleeding continues. The Ministry of Health doctors decided they could trust the pregnant woman herself to diagnose and treat hemorrhage instead of training the village midwife.

It turns out that women liked the idea of misoprostol in their pocket because it helped them feel a little more in control of an unpredictable situation: Will I go into labor at night? Is the doctor available? Will the hospital be open? Do I have transportation? Women received much more information than normal during their prenatal visits (about other danger signs and what to do in case of problems), and study results[46] of the Indonesia intervention with misoprostol showed that more women and their husbands tended to look for a hospital or clinic to give birth instead of staying at home with the bidan de desa.

The study also showed that women took the pills correctly, and that a large proportion of the women reported they would be willing to use misoprostol in their next pregnancies, pay for it themselves, and recommend it to friends.[47] What a relief for women and their families to know that someone, somewhere, is concerned enough about their welfare to allow them to take a pill without having a doctor's prescription. What a relief for the doctors to know that they don't have to connect with the traditional midwives anymore – that women can be their own health care professionals when the "real" one is not around. What a relief to see the maternal mortality rate from hemorrhage dropping in Indonesia...oh, sorry. That didn't happen.

After all the hundreds of studies involving the effectiveness of misoprostol for preventing postpartum hemorrhage, scientists have come to the same conclusion: it's better than a placebo (nothing) but not as good as injectable oxytocin (mother nature's own hormone to contract the uterus). They don't bother to mention, of course, that preventing anemia in the first place would probably help reduce the incidence of hemorrhage in childbirth. Or that training the bidan de desa to use oxytocin correctly for preventing postpartum hemorrhage would probably help reduce maternal deaths dramatically. No one, not even a trained physician, has time to get a hemorrhaging woman to a hospital if that woman is giving birth at home – and that's where most mothers prefer to give birth.

But wait a minute. Who discovered that an anti-ulcer pill to stop stomach bleeding (common registered trademark names are Tagamet, Cytotec, Arthrotec, Oxaprost, Cyprostol, Mibetec, Prostokos, or Misotrol) could be used by postpartum women to help stop *uterine* bleeding? How did doctors discover that *vaginal* insertion of misoprostol works on a first trimester uterus to cause contractions strong enough to expel unwanted "products of conception" (thus a safe, clean, and effective abortion)? And how did they determine that vaginal misoprostol opens up a closed, nine-months-pregnant cervix to stimulate contractions and artificially begin labor?

The active ingredient in misoprostol and all those anti-ulcer medications is prostaglandin. Midwives have known about prostaglandins for centuries as a natural substance that will soften a cervix – it's in the primrose plant and also in sperm, which is why midwives have always recommended that a woman past her due date have sexual intercourse with her partner to soften her cervix.

Technically, prostaglandins are hormones, although they are classified chemically under the name of "fatty acids." They have enormous physical effects on the body, just like hormones. The name "prostaglandin" derives from the prostate gland. When it was discovered by a Swedish scientist in 1935, in semen, he attributed the gooey liquid to prostate secretions, even though it came from the seminal vesicles.[48]

Prostaglandins act in various ways on various cells, such as smooth muscle cells, causing constriction or dilation; on platelets, causing them to bunch together for clotting or to fall apart for bleeding; and on spinal neurons, causing pain. Prostaglandins have a wide variety of actions, including contracting muscles and reducing inflammation. Other effects include calcium movement in and out of cells, hormone regulation, and cell growth control. Among their many pharmacological effects, they:

- Contract the uterus
- Prevent the closure of ductus arteriosis in premature babies' hearts
- Prevent and treat peptic ulcers
- Dilate blood vessels to help treat Reynaud's disease (blood flow to the extremities)
- Help treat pulmonary hypertension
- Help treat glaucoma
- Help treat penis erection problems

Misoprostol – the synthetic name for prostaglandin – *is not licensed for use in labor* either in the US or in the UK, but it is widely used "off-label" to induce labor by softening the cervix and stimulating uterus contractions. Potential side effects of vaginally inserted misoprostol include severe cramping, hyper-stimulation of the uterus resulting in fetal heart rate increase, and there are reports of uterus rupture – with the fetus still inside the uterus. While women are only now beginning to hear about the serious adverse effects of this drug, obstetricians are still enthusiastic. At a recent conference an obstetrician said, "This is a lovely drug – it gets the women delivered really quickly."

For decades the Federal Drug Administration of the United States government prohibited pharmaceutical companies from condoning misoprostol in any way for obstetric or gynecological use. The pharmaceutical companies didn't want the legal headache of promoting a drug that hadn't been FDA approved. They also didn't want to shoulder the costs of manufacturing, packaging, and distributing a dedicated misoprostol product to obstetrics (instead of its legal dedication to ulcers).[49] The conclusion of a pharmaceutical company representative in an October 2003 Gyunity Health Projects meeting was that "Under ordinary circumstances, it is not financially feasible or desirable to market a dedicated misoprostol product for reproductive health indications. Furthermore, it is likely that even if a dedicated product is made available, hospitals that routinely stock Cytotec® will still use it for reproductive health indications due to its lower cost."[50]

Beverley Beech of the Association for Improvements in the Maternity Services (United Kingdom) writes in an editorial in 2006[51] about misoprostol and how Searle, the drug company that manufactures it, was "advised" by the FDA to write a warning letter to consumers about its use in reproductive health. Searle merely noted that they did not recommend or condone misoprostol for use in pregnancy or childbirth because there were (at that time) "no scientific studies on the subject."

In 2006 the Cochrane Data Base (the "gold standard" for summaries of scientific research in medical fields) published the following statement about their review of several studies done on the obstetric use of misoprostol:[52]

> The increase in uterine hyper-stimulation with fetal
> heart rate changes [when using misoprostol] is a
> matter for concern. The studies were not sufficiently
> large to exclude the possibility of uncommon
> serious adverse effects. The increase in meconium
> stained liquor [when the amniotic fluid contains
> feces from the distressed fetus] also requires further
> investigation. Misoprostol (Cytotec) cannot be
> recommended for routine use for labour induction
> at this stage. It is also not registered for such use in
> the US.

And yet misoprostol is used by obstetricians to induce labor in every hospital in every country. I repeat: *everywhere.*

Financial priorities aside, one wonders why medical professionals invest so much effort in this ingenious use for a stomach ulcer drug. It may have something to do with control over a frightening situation – natural childbirth. With misoprostol, the doctor can control the time and the contractions and the delivery and even the hemorrhage after the delivery. It's as if he were in charge of the birth.

In her debate with obstetricians about misoprostol use for inducing labor, Henci Goer wonders in a *Midwifery Today* article,[53] "What's in it for the obstetrician?" In her article she writes about how a disinformation campaign by obstetricians and gynecologists is done "with forethought and malice." She writes:

> On the principle that "the best defense is a good
> offense," the American College of Obstetricians
> and Gynecologists (ACOG) decided that it would
> take a leaf from the book of other industries' image
> or litigation problems. Like cigarette companies,
> formula companies and the manufacturers of unsafe
> cars, it would run a Public Relations campaign. This
> campaign had two arms:
>
> • Sell the public on the idea that obstetricians are
>   heroes, selflessly doing their best against diffi-

cult odds to safeguard the health and well-being and protect the interests of women and babies. Anyone who criticized or tried to rein in obstetric management then became the villains in the piece.

- Co-opt the research so that it could be used as a bastion within which obstetricians could continue business as usual. What is true in the popular press is equally true in the professional literature: If you "talk the talk," few will look behind the façade to see the weaknesses in logic or reasoning.

What about these editorials? They are usually comments on studies published within prestigious, peer-reviewed medical journals. However, if one takes the time to read the studies carefully, one will notice the obvious flaws.

In the case of using misoprostol to induce labor, the FDA *prohibited* its use in reproductive health. Period. A 2001 study published in the *New England Journal of Medicine*[54] admits, if you read the entire content and not just the conclusions, adverse effects of misoprostol for labor induction. The authors note that whether misoprostol or oxytocin is used to induce labor, high cesarean rates are the same result.

"However," the authors of the study concluded, "there is ... strong and consistent evidence to support the use of misoprostol ... for induction of labor." The accompanying editorial, signed by two official representatives of ACOG, chastised Searle, the drug's manufacturer, and the FDA for opposing misoprostol use. "The real victims," the editorial stated, "are pregnant women who receive treatment in hospitals that will not allow the use of misoprostol. Alternative medications are expensive and relatively ineffective." (This statement contraindicated their own study results!) The editorial went on to ask the FDA to "recognize the beneficial roles misoprostol can have," and closes with: "Women in the United States should not be deprived of access to misoprostol."

Let's look at this. According to the FDA,[55] misoprostol can cause, among other things, "uterine tetany [a massive and painful contraction like tetanus] with marked reduction of blood flow to the fetus, uterine rupture sometimes requiring hysterectomy, amniotic fluid embolism [like a blood clot causing stroke or death], severe genital bleeding, shock, fetal bradycardia [slow heartbeat for the fetus], and fetal and maternal death. Uterine hyper-stimulation may increase the incidence of meconium [when the stressed fetus poops inside the womb] and cesarean delivery." Yet the good doctors at the *New England Journal of Medicine* decided that "women should be given the opportunity to have their baby when and where they want." Of course, that doesn't mean at home, with their family, or when natural contractions dictate....

That misoprostol article in the *Journal* was instrumental in the FDA's decision to retract its own science-based ban. Interestingly, though, the grounds weren't reassurance for misoprostol safety. According to Reuters,[56] "The contraindication and certain precautionary wording have been removed to reflect the fact that the drug is widely used to induce labor and delivery." In other words, the FDA decided to let obstetricians use misoprostol *because they were already using it*. In fact, as noted above, the package insert still details the horrific things that can happen when women are given misoprostol to induce labor, but now the list is buried on page eight, and the warning icon of a pregnant woman with a circle and slash is gone.

If misoprostol is as common and wonderful as doctors make it out to be, why are there so many legal restrictions for its use in the public marketplace? Well, because it causes uterine contractions, and women could use it willy-nilly to provoke an abortion, that's why! And why in this world would anyone want to have control over a woman's baby-making abilities, except the woman herself? Because sometimes the baby-making ability is forced upon her, as we'll see in the next true story – only one of millions of stories that happen around the world every day.

Pregnant Pause

Obstetric Myths About Labor
Induction and Conduction

Reader, this is quite a long Pregnant Pause. Let's consider this pause like the pushing stage...sometimes it just takes longer; especially if you are on your back, haven't eaten all day long, are exhausted, and you're being yelled at by people behind purple masks, crying, "Push it out!"

Myth #1: A woman has 40 weeks to gestate a baby to term. If she passes 40 weeks, she needs to be "induced" to begin labor – ready or not – because a "late term" baby has more "risks."

Whether or not to induce labor is based on a false premise. Franz Karl Naegele, the doctor who made up the rule about 40 weeks, was born July 12, 1778 in Dusseldorf, Germany. He determined the "average" length pregnancy based on an "average" menstrual cycle of 28 days. Thus, counting from the first day of the last menstrual period (10 x 28 days), a "normal" gestation takes 10 lunar months or 280 days. Some women do know when their last period occurred; many do not. Most women don't have a 28-day cycle, and many women have a different cycle every month depending on stress, food intake, disease, or disaster. Middle- and upper-class black women, poor women of any race, or poorly nourished women have much shorter or much longer cycles than 28 days.

Medical professionals responded, of course, to the *hundreds* of scientific studies saying that gestation dates depend on race, class, and country of origin:[57] they decided to promote fetal ultrasound to determine dates; then induce if she was "past dates."

Myth #2: An ultrasound in the first trimester accurately determines fetal gestational age.

Ultrasounds are known to have a margin of error of +/- 5 days in the first trimester, eight days in the second, and up to *22 days margin of error* in the third trimester![58] In a more recent Danish study,[59] the median prediction errors estimated by sonography in the first and second trimesters and by corrected LMP (last menstrual period) according to cycle length were 2.32, 0.16, and 3.00 days, respectively, in women with certain LMP, and 1.71, 0.00, and 3.00 days, respectively, in women with uncertain LMP.

Ultrasound may be a prediction for due dates – if the mother has access to ultrasound – but the real point is: Why are doctors inducing women's labors and conducting women's birthing process in the first place?

Myth #3: A woman in labor has a certain number of hours to get the baby out.

This number is based on Friedman's Curve (developed by Milton Friedman in 1954). If she doesn't have the first stage of labor within a certain time frame, labor must be induced. If she doesn't push the baby out during the second stage within a certain time frame, forceps must be used or a C-section is warranted.

First of all, epidural anesthesia lengthens labor time. Second, *many* studies done by midwives and nurses around the world argue that the length of time depends on too many factors (including presence or absence of the woman's partner or her midwife); that race, nutrition, and fear play a big role in labor; and that induction of labor has many side effects – not the least of which is hyper-stimulation of the uterus with many attendant problems. (See Pub-Med online for around 400 studies on this topic: www.ncbi.nlm. nih.gov/entrez.)

The average length of labor for first-time mothers (primi-gravida) and many-times mothers (multi-gravida) for white women in the US today is similar to the average length of labor described by Friedman in 1954. However, in one racially and economically mixed-patient study,[60] a wider range of "normal" occurred. First time mothers remained in the first stage of labor for up to 26 hours and the second stage of labor up to 8 hours with no adverse effects to mother or infant. Multi-gravida mothers remained in the first stage of labor for up to 23 hours and the second stage of labor for up to 4.5 hours with good birth outcomes.

CHAPTER 8

Who's in Charge?

Nine-year-old Cecilia[61] hadn't even known she was pregnant at first. She thought she was throwing up every morning and not eating because she had swallowed river water that time she and her cousins went swimming. She didn't know why her stomach hurt so much if she wasn't eating – unless she had parasites again. That had happened before. But her auntie, Tía Susie, soon discovered Cecilia's morning sickness, her paleness, and her desire to stay in the kitchen instead of playing with her cousins. Tía Susie advised Cecilia's mother, Carmen, that her daughter might be pregnant. And Carmen sat her daughter down at the small kitchen table one day after school, hot tea and a plate of tortillas shared between them. Every mother's nightmare.

"We need to have a talk, *mi amor*," she said to her daughter. They had never even spoken about menstruation before, but they talked of missing a period now.

Cecilia, with her thick brown hair tied in a ponytail, nut-brown skin from playing outdoors, and chewed fingernails, lived in a small Nicaraguan town surrounded by coffee-growing mountains. She belonged to the Catholic parish of San Juan and had received her First Holy Communion from Father Francisco. She walked to her fifth grade class at the parochial school every day. She wore her uniform proudly because she knew her mother worked extra nights sewing to earn enough money to send her to that school with that uniform.

Cecilia knew what pregnancy meant, of course. She just didn't understand why it had happened to her. She never wanted sex with her uncle – but he did with her. Children in Nicaragua – and in most countries, both boys and girls – often have no information about sex and no choice about when, how, or with whom they will have sexual relations. Sex education in schools had been introduced in Nicaragua during the 1980s under Daniel Ortega's Sandinista government. The Ministry of Education had had classes and textbooks about biology and sex for all school-aged children, but that all changed with the election of president Violeta Chamarro in 1992. She was a very conservative Catholic, as were her appointed Ministers of Health and Education, and they removed sex-ed from the school curriculum.

By 2002, when Cecilia was in third grade, a different Minister of Education had boldly proposed *Education for Life,* a sex-education manual for seventh and eighth graders attending Nicaragua's public schools. The professors from the Ministry wanted to encourage conversations among teachers, parents, and students about self-esteem, self-respect, the human body, emotions, affection, love, sexual relations, prevention of sexually transmitted diseases, and prevention of pregnancy. But the manual never got distributed and those classes were never taught. Powerful evangelical Christian and Catholic groups opposed the manual and labeled it as "libertine," "lacking Christian ethics," and "promoting promiscuity."[62] Their media attacks and threats of countrywide strikes led the education minister to withdraw the manual.

So Cecilia and her classmates in Nicaragua did not benefit from sex education in school. Instead, like far too many unsuspecting children in Nicaragua, they learned about sex from men who believe they can cure AIDS or venereal disease if they have sex with a virgin. Or they learned about sex from men who believe they can avoid venereal diseases if they have sex with a virgin. Or who believe their right as a man dictates that they can have sex with whomever they want, whenever they want. Or from men who are unaccustomed to think about the person they have sex with at all – they just think about having sex. The Nicaraguan government's Women's Commission[63] estimated that in 2003, twenty percent of sexual crimes in the country were committed against girls under age thirteen. It said sixty percent of those crimes were committed by fathers, stepfathers, or grandfathers, or – in Cecilia's case – an uncle.

The day after that tear-filled table talk about menstruation and pregnancy, Carmen had spoken with the local police office to report that her daughter had been raped. The investigating officer had demanded to know why Cecilia had "allowed that to happen." After that humiliation, Carmen had taken her daughter to their family physician for an examination. The doctor shook his head and said, "Yes, your daughter is about six weeks pregnant, but she has no diseases that I can detect." And before long, the local radio reporter had heard the news and tried to question little Cecilia; but Carmen and Tía Susie didn't allow it. By later that week, Cecilia's mother, her aunts, the police, the reporter, and eventually the entire community, all had looked to the doctor for advice: "Well? What do we do now?"

The doctor had pronounced Cecilia too young to carry the child to full term, that her body and hips would never be able to survive the complications of a pregnancy or birth, that she faced a threat of hemorrhage from a spontaneous abortion, and that her life was in danger.

"She must have a therapeutic abortion," declared the man of medicine. "But I can't do that here," he added. "You'll have to travel to Managua and get permission from a panel of doctors." (At that time in Nicaragua, anyone who wanted an abortion had to get permission from a panel of three doctors, and those doctors decided what to do based upon legislation saying that therapeutic abortion was illegal unless the life of the mother was threatened.) A six-hour bus trip from their village to Managua was too far for Cecilia and her mother and aunt, and too expensive. Plus, they didn't know any doctors there, let alone one who would perform an abortion.

By now Cecilia's parish priest, Father Francisco, had heard the news and made pronouncements from the pulpit and on public radio about the murderous crime of abortion. The Nicaraguan wire services picked up the story. Television news cameras showed up in the little mountain town the very next week. Carmen and Tía Susie wouldn't let anyone talk with Cecilia. Cecilia didn't want to talk with anyone. As far as she was concerned, she was dying of embarrassment and shame and couldn't die from the complications of pregnancy or childbirth soon enough.

The Catholic Church rigorously, loudly, and publicly denounces all abortion in Latin American countries. In this culture, the priest, the doctor, or the government official obligingly take on burdensome paternal responsibilities. These "father figures" are trusted to know what's best for the weak, for those who need protection. While there were undoubtedly some who had sincere concerns about saving the life of an unborn child, in the passion of their crusade they had forgotten the life of another little child; that of innocent, 9-year-old Cecilia. Struggling with the aftermath of rape, then public humiliation, she was now facing the possibility of her own death. The priests could not ask themselves the question, "What would I be doing if this were my own child?"

Father Francisco dutifully granted all interviews concerning the straying sheep named Cecilia. The Bishop of Managua threatened anyone involved in an abortion for Cecilia would be excommunicated – including Cecilia, who had received her First Holy Communion just that year.

Physicians are trained to name a fetus "the product of conception" and to assume responsibility for the health and well-being of the unborn, a responsibility determined by a code of ethics from Hippocrates (whose mother was a famous Athenian midwife, by the way). Abortion had been illegal in Nicaragua for more than a century, punishable by prison terms of up to four years for women undergoing the procedure and ten years for doctors who performed it. Then, on November 2 of 2006, Nicaragua's legislature voted to ban all abortions, eliminating even long-standing exceptions for rape, malformation of the fetus, and risk to the life or health of the mother.[64] Nicaragua's tight presidential elections in 2006 offered the country's anti-abortion movement the opening it had been waiting for: with ex-Sandinista, now born-again-Evangelical Christian presidential candidate Daniel Ortega suddenly showing his conservative bent, and other conservative opposition parties evenly divided, none of the top three candidates could afford to alienate the Catholic or Evangelical churches – or the legislators. (A side story: in March 1998, Zoilamerica Narvaez publicly accused her stepfather, former President Daniel Ortega, of having sexually abused her from the age of eleven. As a member of the National Assembly, Ortega claims parliamentary immunity and has refused to stand trial.)

According to the *Washington Post*[65] and other press stories, every major medical society in Nicaragua opposed the abortion ban proposal before the Nicaraguan legislature. Their concerns were echoed by Nicaragua's health minister and a long list of foreign embassies and international organizations, such as the United Nations. But the Nicaraguan legislators wouldn't even meet with doctors. Imagine, the country's three most powerful representatives, all men, in a fight over who owns rights over a woman's own body and her own fetus.

But stricter abortion laws have not prevented young women from seeking a termination of their pregnancy – legal or not. Recently the director of the Berta Calderon hospital, the largest public hospital in the nation, reported that botched abortions were filling half the hospital's fifty obstetrics beds at any given time. He complained that much of the hospital budget was being spent to save the lives of young girls who had had an illegal abortion.

"Unsafe, illegal abortions are among the leading causes of death for Nicaraguan women," says Dr. Ana Maria Pizarro, a gynecologist who directs the *Si Mujer* health center in Managua. She says a government study in 1998 estimated that 36,000 illegal abortions a year were performed in this country of five million people.[66, 67]

While Cecilia's story made headlines in 2002 because of her very young age, Nicaraguan adolescents and their extremely high pregnancy rates rarely make headlines. According to a 2004 Inter-Hemispheric Resource Center publication, *twenty-seven percent* of all female Nicaraguan adolescents are either pregnant or have given birth. This is the highest adolescent fecundity rate in all Latin America. One of every three females who dies from a childbirth-related complication in Nicaragua is a teenager. In Nicaragua, conservatives within the Ministries of Health and Education, along with Vatican representatives, dictate who receives family planning methods or information – and who receives an abortion when family planning fails.

Two weeks after Carmen and Cecilia had had their eye-opening experiences in their hometown, they traveled with Tía Susie to Managua and begged doctors at hospitals all over the city for an abortion. They had raised money for the bus trip and the abortion by selling household items and receiving donations from neighbors. Since that table talk two weeks previously, Cecilia had become front-page news in every paper, magazine, radio broadcast, and TV talk show from Argentina to Mexico. The debate was never about Cecilia, of course, but about the Rights of the Fetus versus the Right of the Woman to Abort the Fetus. What about the right of Cecilia to live?

Some had asked, "What about the rights of the father to his child?" Cecilia's uncle expressed no interest. The authorities did not threaten him with arrest for raping his niece, nor for having sex with a minor. And the uncle demonstrated enough sense not to ask for paternal rights to his child – the one growing inside the other child. He escaped to Mexico City.

Cecilia, Carmen, and Tía Susie finally found a sympathetic woman doctor who performed the ten-minute procedure to remove the "products of conception" in March of 2003. Cecilia suffered no bleeding or infection. The three returned to their village in the mountains and life went on, except that Cecilia was not welcomed back to the flock at San Juan Catholic Church or the parochial school. She was excommunicated, as were her mother, her aunt, and the doctors and the nurses at the clinic where the simple suction procedure was performed.

Cardinal Miguel Obando y Bravo of the Archdiocese of Nicaragua is now retired, but very active in politics with Archbishop Fernando Saenz Lacalle of El Salvador where, in 1998, lawmakers removed all exceptions to that nation's ban on abortion and increased penalties to up to 50 years' imprisonment. Cardinal Obando y Bravo announced that those involved in Cecilia's abortion had "excommunicated themselves" under church law. (He never threatened excommunication for the uncle.) According to BBC news reports at that time, the Cardinal's statement prompted tens of thousands of women in Nicaragua – and supporters in Europe – to sign petitions demanding to be excommunicated themselves.

Passions were so inflamed that Central American Catholic bishops issued an open letter comparing abortions to terrorist bus bombs. Those burning "bus bomb" passions in the year of Cecilia's near-death-experience also resulted in the Minister of Health resigning her post. If the "threat" posed by one nine-year-old girl is enough to wreak havoc among Nicaragua's religious and political leaders, could the power held by those leaders need further examination?

As of this writing, another young girl now threatens conservative convention in Nicaragua by asking for a legal abortion. She is eleven years old and eight weeks pregnant. Health Minister Jose Alvarado said in a local television interview that the government's Ministry of the Family is in charge of the case and has custody of the child. He said a panel of officials will determine whether this eleven-year-old rape victim should give birth. My midwife friends and I wonder whether that panel of officials with authority over this life and death consists of priests and doctors, or of mothers and aunts.

Who are these people claiming cultural authority in any given country? It depends on the power structures and also how authority is perceived. Psychologist and author Jeanne Achterberg says that the cosmology of a culture determines who assumes positions of leadership. Cosmology comes from the Greek words *cosmos* (the Universe) and *logos*, or discourse: that is, the study of the Universe in its totality, and by extension, humanity's place in it. She writes in *Woman as Healer*[68] that "almost always those individuals [who assume leadership] must have the face of god(s). Since the vocation of healer, particularly, is associated with the sacred, and the healing beliefs of any culture directly reflect the nature of the gods, only in those times when the reigning deity has had a feminine, bisexual, or androgynous nature have women been able to exercise the healing arts with freedom and power." While god has a man's face, then man (and masculinity – bereft of the feminine and all that implies) becomes the authoritative power.

In the next chapter we'll see why authority depends on the situation, and not necessarily on who has authoritative knowledge.

Pregnant Pause

RITUAL AND REASON

The following summarizes the rituals, taboo or customs of pregnancy and birth found among **all indigenous American peoples** from Alaska to Antarctica, with very few variations, and the corresponding reason or purpose. Remember, these First People have been around for a few thousand years and have developed these belief systems based on experience and legends. When teaching traditional midwives or women and families from any culture, but particularly the Americas, we must always be mindful of how their traditions will effect their learning or compliance to our birthing expectations.

Ritual -   The pregnant woman must be careful not to sit with her back toward the sun while outdoors.

Reason -   Because if the pregnant woman's back gets too warm, it may cause the placenta to stick there and not come out.

Ritual -   Pregnant women should no attempt any knitting or embroidery while pregnant.

Reason -   Knitting or sewing may cause the umbilical cord to become tangled around the baby.

Ritual -   Blood has to accumulate in all parts of the body, especially the uterus, to make a strong baby. Thus, edema of the hands, face, or feet is a good thing.

Reason -   Since the first sign of pregnancy is when menstruation doesn't occur, it naturally means blood is accumulating in the body to make a new baby.

Ritual -   The pregnant woman must avoid hot foods and fires or becoming too warm in the sun.

Reason -   Heat favors the elements of down and out, which may provoke an unwanted abortion. Cold elements are better to maintain the pregnancy.

Ritual -   During labor the woman should drink hot teas made from oregano, rosemary, orange flower, or carrot greens.

Reason -   These herbs are natural contracting agents for the uterus, and are also hot elements, which stimulate down and out motions necessary for birth.

Ritual -   During birth, the woman must avoid air currents, thus maintaining a warm and humid environment.

Reason -   Heat and warmth favor the exit (down and out) of the baby, the placenta, and the "dirty" blood that has been accumulating for nine months. Cold elements are taboo during the birth (like a cold, sterile hospital room).

Ritual -   The placenta (considered to be the child's twin) must be washed and buried by the husband in a secret, shady place.

Reason -   If this ritual is not performed correctly, the mother or baby may become very sick or even die, as the placenta has its own spirit.

Ritual -   During the postpartum, the mother should avoid bathing or washing in any manner.

Reason -   Water is a cold element and may interfere with the exit of the "dirty blood" that has been accumulating.

Ritual -   During the first three days of life, the newborn is given anise tea instead of colostrum from the mother' breast.

Reason -   Anise tea, along with some urine from the eldest
            brother of the newborn, are very good for cleansing
            the intestines of the baby.

Ritual -   Colostrum, the first milk, must be expressed by the
            mother and tossed out.

Reason -   Colostrum, which is the same color as pus, is consid-
            ered "dirty" and the cause of colic, making the baby
            cry more.

CHAPTER 9

Does Authority Matter?

Anthropologists study humanity. They observe silently, take notes, remain objective. When they finally publish results of their quiet examinations, the consequences may be startling, enlightening, or even threatening to the people and practices they have scrutinized. But the results usually are not disputed, because they are so objective! Anthropologists just tell it like they see it, with those poker faces of theirs, and when the fires start raging they say, "I'm just the messenger; I'm not the one who started the fire, fanned the flames, or called the emergency crews. I'm just taking notes; I don't intervene, I interview."

Medical anthropologists study systems of medical knowledge and health care relating to healers and those healed. Medical anthropology combines social sciences like art, psychology, and sociology with biological sciences like anatomy, physiology, and chemistry. These Ph.D. doctors may observe and comment upon the patient/practitioner relationship, environmental or social factors affecting health and illness, and the impact of bio-medical technologies on people.[69] They speak with authority because they are very strict about their code of ethics as *observers* of phenomena – they don't implement or intervene, just watch, interview, record, and narrate. For example, medical anthropologists observe that traditional societies treat birth as an expression of health rather than sickness.

Which is why, when medical anthropologists get together and have a conference or write a book about childbirth and authoritative knowledge, the rest of us should sit up and pay attention – because their observations reflect our canary-in-the-coal-mine behaviors concerning health and sickness.

The term *Authoritative Knowledge* (AK) comes from anthropology and sociology. Robbie Davis-Floyd and Carolyn Sargent write in their book, *Childbirth and Authoritative Knowledge,*[70] that AK is used to describe how a particular system of knowing exists among a group of peers, and that by their consensus, it carries more weight than other systems of knowing.

For example, master plumbers have more authoritative knowledge over apprentice plumbers. Editors have more AK than journalists, who have more than writing students. And in her community, the traditional midwife has more authoritative knowledge than the mother giving birth. She even has more authoritative knowledge than the young university-graduated nurse or doctor in her village, because the "professional" is an unknown entity among her group of peers, which is her community. Authoritative knowledge is all about accountability in a community of practice – *not that the knowledge is correct, but that it matters.* Just as certain medical practices based on bad habits or fear may be incorrect, it still matters that other professional health providers believe those practices are correct.

A case in point: millions of women around the world today receive a senseless surgical incision during childbirth upon the most tender and private part of their body – in Eastern or esoteric models, upon the basic first chakra – called an episiotomy, a cut on her perineum, just as the head of her baby is about to be born. According to doctors and midwives trained in the medical model (their authoritative knowledge in their community of practice) the episiotomy has always been "necessary". Now, after fifteen years and hundreds of scientific studies on thousands of women showing that "necessity" to be false, in fact harmful, why do doctors and midwives continue this barbaric practice? Because again, authoritative knowledge is all about accountability in a community of practice – *not that the knowledge is correct, but that it matters.*

Anthropologists will tell us that this episiotomy ritual, or custom, is based on fears from medical anecdotes. The fear, generated by antique medical men not knowing women's anatomy, believed the baby's head would "get stuck" or that "brain damage" may occur because of the force of the tiny cranium against the pelvis. In fact, the cranium of the baby, along with the force of uterine contractions, opens up the cervix (not the pelvis, a bony structure which is opened up by hormones during pregnancy) so the baby can be born. Birth had been accomplished this way for a hundred million years before doctors invented episiotomies. That cutting ritual occurred around the same time that the "laying on your back to give birth" ritual occurred. Physically, it's almost impossible to push a baby out while flat on your back; thus, the episiotomy. Throughout history women have always given birth in the squatting position. But of course the vertical position, a position where the woman is physically *above* the doctor, doesn't accommodate the doctor's demeanor or comfort.

The ritual of female genital cutting in many African cultures becomes another startling example of authoritative knowledge influencing behavior because it matters and not because it's healthy. This mutilation – the reasons for which, let alone the act, are difficult for those of us not accustomed to the ritual to understand – is described by social psychologist Hanny Lightfoot-Klein in her report about cutting away the labia majora, minora, and clitoris of girls:[71]

> Horrendous pain, massive bleeding and raging infection may be expected to result from the procedures themselves, which are still carried out in the majority of cases without even local anesthesia. Normal passage of urine and menstrual blood are rendered all but impossible by infibulation, a sewing up of the vaginal orifice, down to a match stick sized opening, after the child's clitoris and labia have been cut away. Urinary and menstrual debris

accumulating behind this "chastity belt of skin and
scar tissue" create a perfect breeding ground for
infection. Events such as defloration and childbirth,
when these infibulations must be forcibly torn or cut
open, are once again fraught with pain, infection,
and almost inevitably, massive and often fatal blood
loss.

This ritual, done under the sponsorship of the *women* in a
family, involves traditional midwives or grandmothers who have
the authoritative knowledge and experience in their community of
practice. I have read many reports about, and have known many
women who have had, this hideous maiming; they explain that it's
done to maintain cleanliness, uphold a woman's virtue, and sustain
her virginity until her husband "claims" her for his own.

Breathe.

Now think about all the reasons male circumcision rituals
involve authoritative knowledge in a community of practice – also,
not because it's right, but because "it matters." Lightfoot-Klein goes
on to note that once we get past the "it's only skin" argument for the
mutilation, people could concentrate on the genitalia structures
and how that genital mutilation affects sexual function over the
life of the maimed person.

She writes, "The 'It's only a little piece of skin, the woman does
not miss it' argument loses out very quickly with men when they are
informed that the clitoris is analogous to the penis, and how would
they feel about having 'just a little piece' of their penis removed.
By the same token, removal of the male foreskin is functionally
analogous to removal of the female labia, whose function is to
protect the clitoris and to keep it moist. The mere thought of an
unprotected and dry clitoris would make any woman cringe. It is
also highly unlikely that such a clitoris would have retained much
of its original sensitivity by the time a woman reaches the age of
thirty."[72]

As all home birth midwives know, childbirth can be a very
sexual – even orgasmic – experience for the physically, emotionally,
or spiritually non-maimed woman. Yes, I said sexual and not (just)

sensual. This sexuality, made manifest while bringing life into the world, surprised me more than anyone, having been trained and socialized in US hospital procedure, where birth is a medical experience ("for safety reasons") and "sexual childbirth" impossible due to psychic genital mutilation.

Hospital births, which strip the woman of any dignity she may have felt before coming into that institution of illness care, illustrate another sad example of ritual based on AK. The whole point of most hospital rituals are to diminish her and to make her dependent on the authority figures, be it the nurse, the attendant with the wheelchair, the man at the gate with the keys, the midwife, or the doctor. They are the ones with the authoritative knowledge in their community of practice. The pregnant woman or her partner just visit that community.

"Because birth is cultural and historical, it is also political, bound up with the exercise of power," writes Ronald Grimes in his landmark book about ritual and life passages, *Deeply Into the Bone*.[73] Because of the politics and economics involved with birth, some voices are heeded while others are silenced or ignored. Because of fear-based beliefs from press, parents, or peers, mothers and others become subjects of ritualized manipulation during pregnancy and childbirth. Loss of control and fear of chaos underlie countless hospital rituals.

In most cultures we are taught from our first years to earn control and keep it: over our bowels, over our needs and wants, and later over events and our emotions. Think about how we raise little boys to control their emotions, or how we teach female medical students to value their intellect over their intuition. In nursing, midwifery, and medical schools, we are taught to fear tradition and ritual from the unknown world of "patients." We separate the woman from her world, wheel her through the "emergency room," and welcome her into our own world of ritual.

During their prenatal visits, we teach pregnant women how to "gain control" over what we see as a potentially deadly, out-of-control, situation. She is taught to "Let the professionals take care of you...breathe in the Lamaze (or other name) method...pant and push when we tell you and how we instruct you...sit up/lay down/

roll over/go to the bathroom/stay in bed...follow the rules and everything will turn out fine."

Anthropologist Robbie Davis-Floyd argues that hospital procedures serve as rituals because they successfully fulfill important psychological needs:[74]

1. Individual needs of each staff person in the hospital for constant confirmation of the rightness of their technological interventions, and for ways to cope with something not really under their control, which threatens their technocratic model of birth.[75]
2. Individual needs of the woman giving birth for reassurance when faced with the unknown, for "official" recognition by society's designated authorities on birth, and for official confirmation of their belief systems.
3. The important needs of the wider culture to ensure the effective socialization of its citizens and thus society's perpetuation.

This last one has more of an impact than it may seem at first glance. How can simple hospital rituals assure socialization of a citizen? Because vertical authority perpetuates patriarchy. Think about how rituals in any context promote and value conformity within a group. The whole point is control: conformity helps everyone relax around an unknown factor, and it comforts them to count on a vertical line of authority. Congress members and conscripts are two examples.

Membership rituals, years of university medical, nursing, or midwifery school rituals, and hospital rituals that ensure dependency of the patient on the authority figure (doctor, not self) are other examples of how hospital procedures "ensure the effective socialization of its citizens and thus society's perpetuation" based on an authoritative knowledge.

Using a wheelchair to mobilize a healthy pregnant woman is one example of a "purpose-filled" ritual. A pregnant woman demonstrates perfect ambulatory ability when she gets into a car/taxi/bus/donkey-cart or even walks and makes it to the hospital without a wheelchair. We must remember that hospital rituals help personnel reinforce their *assumption* that malfunction may occur at any time, that constant vigilance is necessary to intervene appropriately, and that everyone needs to believe in the technocratic model for it to work.

"To place a healthy woman in a wheelchair instead of allowing her to walk," says Davis-Floyd, "is to tell her that at the very least the hospital thinks of her as disabled and weak." The first impression she makes on the staff, on her husband, and on herself is one of passivity, of helplessness, of fragility. Her lower position encourages the nurses or doctors to talk down to her (literally) or to talk to the standing person at her side. She is seen, and encouraged to see herself, as someone who cannot walk – adding insult to "injury," since walking during labor is one of the most beneficial things a woman can do to ease labor pains and promote regular contractions.

Inserting an IV – with or without the tubes and bags of fluid attached to the IV hub in her arm – becomes one more initiation procedure done in the name of safety and ritual. Others may include removing a woman's own clothes and giving her a hospital gown, shaving her pubic hair, inserting an enema, and separating her from her partner (who is told to leave the woman and "fill out the papers"). These or similar rituals occur in hospitals all over the world, to different degrees. But in almost every case the woman is separated from the one person she trusts most, and must now transfer that trust to a complete stranger who may or may not be sympathetic to her wants and needs. This purpose-filled separation makes her even more dependant on the provider with his authoritative knowledge.

With the magic words "Hospital Policy," two powerful messages appear: first, that the hospital has the *right* to separate the woman from her trusted companion, thus holding higher authority than the family; and second, that the laboring woman belongs to the hospital institution and not to her family unit.

Most fathers in most countries are not allowed into the labor or birthing wards due to lack of privacy – no curtains, no doors, no space between women. (Many places where I've worked have two women to a bed.) In other countries where men may be invited into the "maternity area," fathers become submissive to the women surrounding his partner and especially to the doctors' authority. They lose – or are taught to submit during prenatal classes – their previous role as protector. In some cases, observes anthropologist Sheila Kitzinger, male doctors readily accept the father and form a liaison with him, which, in effect, excludes the woman from making any decisions. Together, the men manage the birth in an aura of male camaraderie.

Kitzinger writes, "Over and over again women's accounts of their birth experiences make it evident that a man's fears were quickly communicated to the woman, and that as well as having to cope with the challenges of her labor, she had to worry about what he was going through."[76] Most fathers don't really understand the need or even want to be present during a birth. Here is a note from a Dad blog[77] about the birth of the couple's third child:

> I know now that alarms on delivery room machines are nothing to fear. Along with smoke detectors and airport security machines, they belong on the long list of devices in American life designed to cry wolf. Apart from that, here is the sum total of what I've learned waiting for my children to be born: 1) arrive sober; 2) do not attempt to be interesting, as it makes the nurses uneasy; 3) never underestimate your own insignificance; and 4) try to get some sleep, as no one else can. Of course, it is important to be present and conscious for the birth of your child. To miss it would be to invite scorn and derision and lead others to speak ill of you behind your back. But up until the moment the child is born, the husband in the delivery room is in an odd predicament. He's been admitted to the scene of the crisis but given no

serious purpose. He's the Frenchman after the war resolution has passed.

In antiquity and throughout the history of humanity, women stayed with a woman to help her go through her transformative process while giving birth, not only to "bring to light" a new life form (Spanish for childbirth is *dar a luz*, literally, to give to the light), but also to give birth to her Self. A girl becomes a woman not just by menstruating, although that is an important life passage, just as is menopause. A woman giving birth connects with all women throughout time. It is this connection that becomes our authority. And women don't have to give birth to understand the connectivity, compassion, and creativity that accompany any of life's transformative processes; growing through any creative or transformative process assures one's own authoritative knowledge, one's inner "knowing." The good news is that men can have this understanding and compassion as well. The bad news is that they often find life-transforming rituals through taking a life, not giving it.[78]

Remember the old joke about choosing a male gynecologist? "Why would you go to a mechanic who never owned a car?" I asked a very good friend of mine, a very compassionate male obstetrician, that very question. He responded, "I don't believe that genitals determine one's ability to relate, to connect, or to accompany. It has more to do with trusting the feminine side of ourselves."

The word midwife means "with woman" and *anyone* who helps another person go through a life-transformative process, connecting to the endless flow of universal energy, remaining true to the feminine and nurturing sides of our selves, knows what it's like to midwife someone. The hospital authority figure is addicted to this life-transforming process for himself.

Even though we all live in a world where science and separation, logic and competition are valued more than intuition, nature, compassion, connection, or emotion, I have more good news: there are many scientific studies showing the value of woman-to-woman support during *any* perceived crisis or life-threatening event. Dr. Laura Klein from Penn State, Pennsylvania, College of Health and Human Development, writes that, "It seems that rather than responding in a fight-or-flight fashion when threatened, fearful or stressed, women may more often tend-and-befriend. Women are more likely to protect and nurture their young, and turn to family and friends for solace when they are stressed."[79]

Remember the physiological characteristics we supposedly have in response to stress, those adrenalin responses we learned in high school biology? Muscles taut, mouth dry, pupils dilated, gut wrenched, and anus tightened, all ready for "fight or flight"? Well, it turns out that all those adrenalin studies from the 1950s were done on young men. In this century, when physiologists and psychologists studied *women* in stressful situations, they discovered that we often react as our female ancestors did when confronted by fire, flood, famine, or fangs: gather the children, group together for protection, and then gab about it with our friends to help calm us all down and process the event (i.e., learn from it).

This new research reiterated that men often react to stress with a traditional fight-or-flight response, and that that response is based on testosterone. Women, on the other hand, manage their stress with a tend-and-befriend response by nurturing their children or seeking social contact, especially with other women, and that response is based on oxytocin and estrogen.

In fact, writes Dr. Klein, when women release the hormone oxytocin in response to stress, it buffers the fight-or-flight response and encourages her to tend to the children and gather with other women. When women engage in this tending or befriending, more oxytocin is released, which further counters stress and produces a calming effect. This calming response does not occur in men, writes Dr. Klein, because testosterone – which men produce in high levels when they're under stress – reduces the effects of oxytocin and gives them the typical fight-or-flight response.[80]

Science also shows us that childbirth becomes safer and easier when mothers are accompanied by other women – particularly when one woman is dedicated to her. In most cultures that would be the traditional midwife. In modern cultures and in hospital settings, that person is usually not the nurse-midwife, the obstetric nurse, or the doctor, but the *doula*.

The term doula, first suggested by anthropologist Dana Raphael,[81] comes from Greek and refers to a woman who personally serves another woman. In the *Journal of Midwifery and Women's Health*,[82] midwives Pascali-Bonaro and Kroeger conclude in their research that "continuous support by a lay woman during labor and delivery facilitates birth, enhances the mother's memory of the experience, strengthens mother-infant bonding, increases breastfeeding success, and significantly reduces many forms of medical intervention, including cesarean delivery and the use of analgesia, anesthesia, vacuum extraction, and forceps." Eleven other randomized controlled studies of women in public hospitals, a place where women normally receive no emotional support, reveal that "companionship by another woman during labor results in mothers needing fewer pain medications, having fewer instrumental deliveries and less Cesarean sections. Babies arrive in better condition at birth, also."[83] Women with laboring woman – it's a good thing.

Why, then, are husbands invited into the delivery room? I believe this practice started because the delivery room in the hospital became masculinized. (It doesn't matter what the genitals of the attending physician or nurse happen to be; it's the system of male-valued intervention instead of female-valued compassion that counts.) When women didn't have anyone to connect with, to trust, or a hand to grip throughout the labor and birth, they naturally wanted the next best thing available – their husbands.

Dr. Keith Ablow, a psychiatrist who treats post-traumatic stress disorders, writes about the recent increase in his practice of husbands who have seen their wives give birth.[84] In the age of the "new man," very little consideration is given to the potentially negative side effects of togetherness in the delivery room.

"Every man I have spoken with over the past few years knows he is expected to be with his wife when his child comes into the world," writes Dr. Ablow. "In the most striking cases, the symptoms that men experience come close to post-traumatic stress disorder, with its roots in the witnessing of an event that involves a threat to the physical integrity of self or others and responding with intense fear, helplessness or horror."[85] (I wonder if it's because in this situation men *cannot* fight or flee that they experience traumatic stress?)

It is miraculous to see a baby's head emerge through the birth canal, but it can also be shocking. It is riveting to see an umbilical cord connecting mother and baby, but it can also be very disturbing. It is exciting to be asked by a doctor to cut that umbilical cord, but also potentially very frightening, even for an otherwise rather fearless man. Dr. Ablow also adds his personal comment about his own wife's births: "I myself recall feeling as if the clinical focus on childbirth during prenatal classes, including the detailed descriptions of the placenta and the meconium, took away from the wonder of the process, rather than adding to it. I don't know what is gained by showing the cross-sectional anatomy of a woman's torso to her lover." But readers, we know: It's not that the practice is correct, but that it matters...and it matters to the authority.

So why do medical doctors want to be obstetricians in the first place? They have no time or inclination to sit around and "be" with women during labor and birth – and less during the postpartum period. (That responsibility goes back into the hands of women relatives or doulas or nurses.) Obstetricians are surgeons. They are trained to intervene, hopefully with a knife, and are taught that technology = chaos control.

I am not suggesting we go backward to high maternal and newborn mortality rates! There is nothing wrong with intervention, antibiotics, surgery, or rescue medicine when it is appropriate. The problem spirals into another kind of chaos when our society values one kind of authority *over* another, one kind of knowing *instead* of another, and interventions as a *substitute* for prevention.

We have seen in this chapter that traditional rituals and practices may not all be beneficial to the health of a pregnant, birthing, postpartum, or lactating woman. We've also seen how rituals based on fear in any culture, including the medical one, may not be beneficial in the long run, even though in the short run they help us feel control over what seems to us a chaotic situation.

Anthropologist Sheila Kitzinger suggests that the real agenda for the medicalization of childbirth is to deny and suppress female sexuality, which obstetricians perceive to be dangerous, threatening, and disruptive.[86] She writes, "By viewing women as defective machines to be managed on the fetus' behalf, by draining the warmth and sensuality out of the experience, by converting it to a time-driven mechanical process, by becoming the central figure in the drama and controlling every aspect of the mother's behavior and activities down to the very sounds she makes, birth comes to feel safe for the doctor." [87]

Kitzinger calls for a midwifery approach: wait and watch. Help women find their own authority, to let them experience this empowering, vital creative force. She emphasizes the female traits of collaboration, compassion, and connection. What I would like to emphasize is that these traits that can be learned; and collaboration, compassion, and connection need not interfere with ritual, science, authoritative knowledge, or even health. These feminine traits may very well enhance advancement in health and in society. Particularly as we set about formulating health care policies, we must remember that health is not the absence of disease, but a reflection of how well we adapt – to our physical, mental, emotional, and spiritual environment, inside and outside of our skin.

Pregnant Pause

Here is an interesting quote from the **World Health Organization** monograph, Having a Baby in Europe. From *Public Health in Europe No. 26*, Copenhagen: Regional Office for Europe, 1985a

"By medicalizing birth, i.e. separating a woman from her own environment and surrounding her with strange people using strange machines to do strange things to her in an effort to assist her (and some of this may occasionally be necessary), the woman's state of mind and body is so altered that her ways of carrying through this intimate act must also be altered and the state of the baby born must equally be altered. The result is that it is no longer possible to know what births would have been like before these manipulations. Most health care providers no longer know what "non-medicalized" birth is. This is an overwhelmingly important issue.

Almost all women in most developed countries give birth in hospitals, leaving the providers of the birth services with no genuine yardstick against which to measure their care. What is the range of length of safe labor? What is the true (i.e. absolute minimum) incidence of respiratory distress syndrome of newborn babies? What is the incidence of tears of the tissues surrounding the vaginal opening if the tissues are not first cut? What is the incidence of depression in women after "non-medicalized" birth? The answer to these, and many more questions is the same: no one knows. The entire modern obstetric and neonatology literature is essentially based on observations of medicalized birth."

CHAPTER 10

What's Love Got to Do With It?

The very first thing I learned during my midwifery training at the Maternidad la Luz Birth Center in El Paso, Texas,[88] was that machines were not used there during labor, birth, or postpartum. The oxygen tank, newborn resuscitation equipment, IV solutions, and other tools of technology were readily available, but they were behind closed closet doors and very rarely called for. Fetal monitoring machines didn't exist at the Center, for example, because we used simple fetoscopes to measure heart rates. We had no electrical equipment at all because, our mentor midwives taught us, mechanical interruptions "stopped the natural flow of a healthy birth." We needed no machines because we were personally present for the mother: our shifts lasted twenty-four hours, every other day. Of the 40 to 50 births a month, only one or two mothers or babies at the Center developed complications and needed referral to the County Hospital a few blocks away. All this information, received during my first visit to the Birth Center in 1990, made my eyebrows go up.

I had worked as a Registered Nurse in many stress-filled US hospitals for twenty-three years: in emergency rooms, operating rooms, and intensive care units for children, adults, and newborns. I knew all about technology and control. Hospital staff are taught

99

that machines help us to prevent complications, or at least help us to intervene when faced with complications, and more importantly, that the person who knows how to run the machine often is the most important person on the "health care" team!

Cesarean rates in all the hospitals where I had worked over the years were about average: 25%. The C-section rate at Maternidad la Luz was 4%. I made the decision to study midwifery at a school within a birthing center and not in a university hospital on purpose. I wanted to learn about birth outside the medicalized model in hospitals and to learn how a woman's own process could possibly be more important or safer than birth based on machines and medical management.

The Maternidad La Luz Birth Center in El Paso began life as an old, rambling three-story wooden house situated on a corner lot near the city center, surrounded by giant chestnut trees. It grew up to be a prenatal and postpartum clinic, a birthing center, and a midwifery school. It has one kitchen for staff and families with a table that seats six; three bathrooms with bathtubs; a garden within the back patio; student classrooms and overnight sleeping rooms in the upstairs attic; and birthing rooms with a double bed in each of the three big bedrooms. The midwives at Maternidad la Luz never said "delivery rooms" – delivery was for pizza, or for Chinese take-out, or for the burritos and tacos from the lady down the alley who made tortillas by hand.

At Maternidad La Luz (and in other birthing centers I have visited that are separate from hospitals) I watched women labor in warm, scented bath waters, or on the outdoor front porch swing, on the toilet, collapsed over my shoulders, or in a rocking chair. A woman gave birth in the bed on her side, sitting up, on all fours, or squatting. Or she gave birth in the water of the tub, or in the garden, or sitting on the toilet, or squatting on top of the gynecological exam table. We midwives kept things clean and convenient. We followed her around with our portable fetoscopes and blood pressure cuffs, thermometers, and sterile instruments. We allowed her to go into a trance wherever and however she needed to do that. We protected her and provided for her – to attend her birth, not deliver her baby.

In a hospital setting, the mother has no time or privacy to go within her most primitive self and allow the natural secretions of oxytocin, progesterone, endorphins, and other hormones to flow effortlessly. And nurses or hospital staff have no time to provide and protect (we are very busy managing our machines...). A laboring woman in a hospital is separated from her partner, her family, and her Self, and society may eventually suffer because of that separation. Published scientific studies now show that interruptions, separations, and manipulations disrupt the natural pulsating flow of oxytocin in the bloodstream, and that this disruption may increase the risks for social problems later in childhood – social problems such as juvenile delinquency, drug addiction, schizophrenia, suicide, or autism disorders. (http://www. birthworks.org/site/primal-health-research.html)

First, let's examine how the natural production and excretion of oxytocin works on the body. Produced in a primitive structure deep within the center of our brains, called the hypothalamus, and stored in the posterior pituitary gland, oxytocin flows into the bloodstream during specific circumstances and in a pulsating fashion. For example, oxytocin released by the pituitary gland in the brains of both partners during intercourse causes contractions of the prostate and seminal vesicles in the male and contractions of the uterus and fallopian tubes in the female. Also secreted during arousal and masturbation, oxytocin affects human sexuality unrelated to procreation: It fills us with feelings of bonding, of euphoria, and of relationship.

And when a mother gets signals from her hungry baby, her oxytocin secretion increases and pulsates liberally into her bloodstream to help with her milk production. During labor the mother, fetus, and placenta all release oxytocin and other hormones – as long as circumstances surrounding that labor and birth don't interrupt that secretion.

Oxytocin is not only produced in the mother's pituitary gland. The fetus *and the placenta* begin secreting oxytocin and directing maternal behaviors even before birth. The process of labor triggers oxytocin release within the brains of both the mother and her fetus, and into their combined circulation via the placenta. Maternal and fetal responses during labor and birth are directed specifically by a placental cortico-tropin-releasing hormone.[89] When this delicate dance of hormones between mother, fetus, and placenta is manipulated – either externally (by interruptions, video cameras, or instructions to the laboring woman) or internally (with sedatives, epidural anesthesia, or IV infusions of synthetic oxytocin) – the manipulations negatively influence oxytocin and other hormone secretion, and it just stops or slows down dramatically.

The medical model is born to manipulate. This model insinuates that pregnancy is an illness; it uses a diagnostic approach to that illness, separates the mind from the body, and emphasizes childbirth as inherently pathological because "something could go wrong, and we are here to fix it." According to the medical model,[90] the doctor is the technician (with machines), the hospital is the factory, and the product is the baby. Even today in medical school, doctors refer to the newborn as the "product of conception." The safety of the fetus (or hospital's liability policy) is pitted against the emotional needs of the mother – as in, "You can't get up to go to the bathroom and unplug the monitor. Do you want your baby to suffer?" Actions are based on the supremacy of technology and importance of science, and only technical knowledge is valued – as in "What does the monitor show?" not "How does the mother feel?" Watch any woman in labor turn her head toward the machine next to her, the machine that the doctor or nurse is fixated on watching, while they pretend to have a dialog between them about the progress of the labor.

According to the medical model, the birth must occur within a certain amount of time. Once labor begins, it should progress steadily within a time frame, and if not, medical intervention is necessary with drugs, forceps, or surgery. Because labor pain is problematic and unacceptable, drugs are made available and encouraged in the medical model. Birth is a service that medicine owns and supplies to society. The obstetrician is the supervisor/manager and skilled technician, who has all the responsibility. The doctor delivers the baby. The doctor determines when, where, and for how long the baby is separated from the mother at birth. The doctor knows best.

How can separation, as opposed to connection, at birth affect long-term socialization? Studies in 1996 from Finland followed more than 11,000 pregnant women and their offspring over ten years.[91] In their sixth or seventh month of pregnancy, the women were asked by investigators whether the pregnancy was wanted, mistimed but wanted, or unwanted. The risk of later schizophrenia was significantly raised for babies born to mothers in the unwanted group compared with the other groups. Schizophrenia can be viewed as an impaired capacity to love, because the personality is separated from its environment.[92]

Another study shows how early separation *together with* rejection by the mother leads to teenage violent crimes. Adrian Raine's team from the University of California at Los Angeles studied 4,269 male subjects born in the same hospital in Copenhagen.[93] They found that the main risk factor for being a violent criminal at age 18 was the association of birth complications with separation and rejection by the mother.

How can manipulation, as opposed to letting go during birth, affect long-term socialization? One study in Sweden published in the *British Medical Journal* looked at the background of 200 opiate addicts born in Stockholm from 1945 to 1966 and took non-addicted siblings as the control group.[94] They found that if a mother had been given certain painkillers during labor, her child was statistically at increased risk of becoming drug addicted in adolescence.

A psychiatrist from Japan, Dr. Ryoko Hattori, evaluated the risks of becoming autistic according to the place of birth.[95] In a long-term retrospective study (looking backwards), she found that children born in a certain hospital were significantly more at risk of becoming autistic. In that particular hospital the routine was to induce labor a week before the expected date of delivery, and to use a complex mixture of sedatives, anesthesia, and analgesics during labor. This practice is very common around the world in all hospitals, not just Japan.

In another case/control study concerning autism, Charlotte Modahl and associates at the Boston University School of Medicine investigated the blood levels of oxytocin in autistic children.[96]

"Despite individual variability and overlapping distribution," writes the team in their published paper, "the autistic group had significantly lower plasma oxytocin levels than the normal group." Also, the oxytocin levels increased with age in the control group but not in the autistic group. In a more recent study from Wayne State University in Detroit in 2001,[97] investigators concluded that oxytocin peptide formation in the neurons is decreased in autistic children, and that these deficits may be important in autism disorders. Why are there no more investigations relating to manipulation of labor, separation at birth, and artificial interruptions with lifelong debilitating conditions like autism disorders in children?

When a woman has no opportunity to be protected, to go within to a primal trance state during birth, to allow her hypothalamus to take over, then all hormonal secretions are thrown off balance. The stress hormones of adrenalin take over sooner than they're supposed to, which happens naturally during the precise moment of pushing out the baby. Stress and fear pump adrenalin into the system during labor, and the body goes into overdrive and high alert: pupils dilate, the mouth and throat dry up, the gut contracts, blood flows to the skeletal muscles instead of the uterus, and panic sets in. The neo-cortex of the brain (the "thinking" and "planning" portion) lights up and takes control. Adrenalin fuels a vicious cycle that leads to fear, more pain, and more adrenalin. Can you imagine having all the lights on, the video camera on, and a crowd of strangers circled around you and your partner in bed making love, shouting "Push! Push! Push!" just as you were both ready to have an orgasm and release oxytocin? Now imagine that scene in the birth room.

Separating mother and baby immediately after birth causes another potentially harmful side effect: oxytocin secretion decreases within each and between both. Yes, between them. When a mother and her newborn gaze into each other's eyes, it stimulates the supra optic nerve bundles – cranial nerves located just behind the eye – which have a direct physiological connection to the posterior pituitary. The pituitary, thus stimulated, secretes oxytocin in both the mother and the baby.[98] Blind mothers (as well as sighted mothers) also recognize and bond with their newborns through the olfactory sensor bulbs (the sense of smell). These nerve bundles also have a "direct hit" on the cranial nerves connected to the pituitary and also cause oxytocin secretion.[99] Oxytocin bathes both bodies, causing natural uterine contractions (to prevent hemorrhage) and allows mothers and their newborns to fall in love with each other. Fathers, grandmothers, and even midwives release a surge of oxytocin while gazing into a baby's eyes, which could very well have a direct impact on bonding, infant protection, and social memory – especially for the father.

Speaking of men and memory, in 2000 Dr. Jan Ferguson and colleagues at Emory University showed that if male mice had their oxytocin-receptor gene altered, they lost their social memory – they could not remember who their nest mates were from one minute to the next.[100] Other memory paths were not affected (they could manage a maze). When the male mice were given injections of oxytocin they could remember their mates for as long as that hormone remained in their bloodstream – even though they didn't carry the receptor gene for oxytocin.

Maternal release of other hormones during childbirth includes endorphins, which act like opiates and may explain how mothers can "forget" some of the pain they suffered during birth. The baby also releases its own endorphins in the birth process, and today there is no doubt that for a certain time following birth, both mother and baby have increased levels of endorphins in their blood. This may assure a "chemical dependency" between mother and newborn, to the benefit of both, and ultimately of the species, by assuring a connection between them.[101]

The second most important thing I learned during my midwifery training at the Birth Center was that childbirth can be an intimate, connecting, sexual experience. This was the midwife's big secret, I thought to myself: Women guide women in rituals of sexual rebirth and transformation. This sexual, sensual experience frightens those of us trained in the medical model of sterility and control.

Within the intimate setting of, say, a bathroom or bedroom at the Birth Center, I sensed I was involved in an ancient initiation ritual during each birth. I felt the grunts and the heat and the spasms and the rhythm and the panting of sexuality during labor.

I heard the same sounds of sex that are so private and taboo in public. I smelled sex from the amniotic fluid, mother's milk, and vaginal secretions, and it permeated our skin. I learned childbirth in this place was juicy, and that "letting go" was promoted instead of counting breaths or maintaining control about when and how the birth should occur. At the Maternidad la Luz Center, the baby slipped out with no episiotomy or forceps, wet and full of life. We dried the eyes-wide-open baby thoroughly, handed it to the mother immediately for skin-to-skin warming to prevent hypothermia, and they continued their bonding with immediate breastfeeding. The newborn stayed with the mother until they both fell asleep – usually within an hour or so. In those pastel-colored rooms, I saw women fall deeply in love with their babies, their partners, the midwives, and especially with themselves. Love was a blessing and birth a force that connected us all.

The entire process was transformative: for me, who learned to let go and be the attendant; for husbands, who witnessed the profound strength of a woman; for the baby, who birthed so awake and alive that sometimes it just sighed and rooted for a breast. The process of childbirth in this way was especially transformative for the woman. It was her birth. We attended. She gave birth to her baby and to her self. One new mother whispered to me while breastfeeding her newborn, "I feel like I am magic. I bring life into being! Look! I am God, at this moment."

Pregnant Pause

Born in the USA

If you think this little book only deals with poor, brown women in far-flung places you will probably never visit, I have a little pause for you to consider. The following information is taken from the Childbirth Connection web site and concerns some fundamental problems with maternity care in the United States.

- The United States is the only wealthy industrialized nation that does not guarantee access to essential health care for all pregnant women and infants. Many women, especially those with low incomes, lack access to adequate maternity care.
- A large body of scientific research shows that many widely used maternity care practices that involve risk and discomfort are of no benefit to low-risk women and infants. On the other hand, some practices that clearly offer important benefits are not widely available in U.S. hospitals.
- Many women, rich or poor, do not receive adequate information about benefits and risks of specific procedures, drugs, tests, and treatments, or about alternatives.
- Childbearing women frequently are not aware of their legal right to make health care choices on behalf of themselves and their babies, and do not exercise this right.

For more information, and to get involved,
see www.childbirthconnection.org

CHAPTER 11

Are We Connecting?

Women healers, or men healers who manage to live with their feminine side intact after education and socialization, aspire to wholeness and harmony with the self, the family, and the community. They see body, mind, and spirit as inseparable and connect "nature" with "human nature." These healers regard sickness as a potential catalyst for growth, and they accompany, lead, teach, and guide others on a path toward health and wholeness. What they don't tend to do is rescue – although they know how to do that. They are inclined to emphasize relationship, links, correlation, and association. These concepts remain diminished or dismissed in medical schools, in hospitals, and in public health policy. We midwives have a saying: If we were Queen, every one of our subjects would live in a safe community, free of poverty, and be loved by their family. Self-respect, dignity, sane public health policy, and healthy mothers with healthy babies, would occur naturally as a result.

Let's look at some of these midwives and hear their stories about connecting science with love, intuition with information, and the art of healing with the courage necessary to outwit the medical model of care.

Barbara in Yemen

Yemen Fun Facts[102]: This very poor country, located south of Saudi Arabia and across the Gulf of Aden from Somalia, gained independence from the Ottoman Empire in 1918. In 2000 the Yemen government determined their border with Saudi Arabia. The capital is Sanaa, the dominant religion is Islam, and the dominant culture is patriarchy. The population of about 21,456,000 lives in an area smaller than France. Of those 21 million, only 70% of the men can read and write and barely 30% of the women can. The national average income per year is about US $900. For every 1,000 babies born, about 60 die before their first month birthday. For every 100,000 live births, 570 women die giving that baby life.

Barbara, a slip of a woman from the mine-pocked mountains of West Virginia, worked in the dusty, bomb-pocked Yemeni town of Saada for seventeen years in the 1980s and '90s.

"It's a walled village with a few gates and a few holes in the wall," she explains. Around town, Barb draped herself in the long, full black "sitaras" that covered her head, face, arms, ankles, and everything in between. During her hospital shift, she wore surgical scrubs that showed off her skinny white, freckled arms, but only within the confines of the labor and delivery room – just one block from her house.

"The walls surrounding Saada are three feet thick, twelve feet high, and made of adobe mud," says Barbara. "For most of the time I lived there, the gates to the village were shut at sunset, so anyone who came to the hospital after sunset had to walk in and get by the guards. From the gate to the hospital was about a fifteen-minute walk. I lived along that route and so I'd often know when I was going to get a call from the hospital to come in, because I would have heard the periodic grunts and cries of a woman in labor as she waddled down the road."

Barbara is a university-trained midwife, with the common sense and loving touch of a traditional healer. Women from all over that part of Yemen came into the hospital to be attended by her and the Dutch midwives who worked as volunteers in the hospital. Barbara and the others learned to speak Arabic. With the women they didn't talk too much, though, just listened and guided during the grunts.

"I lived there during the civil war with South Yemen," Barb says, "and that part of the country was 'Royalist Territory,' meaning we were ruled by warlords who wanted nothing to do with government anything – no health care, no post office, no telephone services, no electricity or road crews – nothing. If any man in our village saw a government worker, he was obliged to shoot him!"

One night she heard a knock on the front door of their house. After dusk nobody walked around visiting and no one ever knocked on their door, so the Dutch midwives and Barb grouped together in a tight, frightened bunch to answer the summons. A man wearing a Yemeni government soldier's uniform, holding his old rifle on one side of him and his in-labor wife on the other, asked for help. The midwives brought him and the woman into the house immediately. If anyone had seen that, they all would have been shot on site.

The midwives decided to hide the husband within their compound, while Barbara accompanied the woman down the dusty road to the hospital. A soldier would never have come into the house of unmarried women, and any Muslim man shouldn't be in a house with any woman inside if he wasn't a relative or married to her. So, they decided, he would be safe inside, while Barbara and the young wife left him there. Barbara noticed, after the wife lifted off her sitara, that the young woman was barely a teenager, shaking and sweating, eyes big as saucers of chocolate sauce.

"I remember she was so very silent during her labor. I told her it was all right to cry out if she wanted. Mostly she just gripped my hand, and even coming from such a thin girl, that grip said more than her cries ever could. Fortunately the baby was born before sunrise, so I could bring mom and babe back to my house, where the husband was able to sneak out of town before he was seen by anyone." Barb attended the birth alone and didn't notify the medical doctor on call that night because the birth was normal, and also because the doctor would have been "obliged" to report that a government soldier had entered the walled city of Saada.

"We had quite a few of those circumstances," she adds lightly. "It was just part of our job, you know, to protect mothers and babies. If we had to protect her husband along the way, well, then we did that too."

Gulalai in Afghanistan

Afghanistan Fun Facts: Ahmad Shah Durrani unified the Pashtun tribes and founded Afghanistan in 1747. The country served as a buffer between the British and Russian empires until it won full independence from British control in 1919. A brief experiment in democracy ended in a 1973 coup and a 1978 Communist counter-coup. The Soviet Union invaded in 1979 to support the tottering Afghan Communist regime, touching off a long and destructive war. With the U.S. and others supporting the opposition (Mujahadeen), many people were killed and entire towns destroyed during the 20-year civil war sponsored by the (at that time) two super powers. When the Taliban took over Kabul and Afghanistan in 1996, they brought stability at last, but at a terrible social price.

The current president, Harmad Karzai, governs about thirty-one million people in a country with the highest mountains and the driest lowlands in Central Asia. Afghanistan has limited natural fresh water resources, inadequate supplies of potable water, soil degradation, overgrazing, deforestation, and desertification, along with air and water pollution. In the midst of this landscape, babies manage to be born, mostly at home, and die at a rate of 160 per every 1,000 born. Maternal mortality clocks in at one of the highest in the world, with about 1,850 dead women for every 100,000 live births – those of whom are counted, of course.

Gulalai is one of many university-trained midwives at the only maternal hospital in the capital, Kabul. I met her at a two-week emergency obstetrics skills course in Bangladesh. Like the other Afghan midwives, Gulalai wore a black, ankle-length galabeya zipped closed up to her neck and a black headscarf tucked tightly under her chubby chin. They all looked like plump penguins or an old-fashioned French nuns when they moved silently down the hallway of the Dhaka General Hospital for their practical skills session in the labor and delivery ward that day.

The Afghan midwives faced the walls of the tiny changing room in the maternity ward and slipped shyly out of their long-sleeved, floor-length galabeya's and headscarves. Exposed before me now in her scrubs for the first time in ten days of training, I noticed Gulalai's short hair, her round body sausaged into the green suit, and her Scandinavian-pale skin. Her shy smile unmasked two big dimples. Her bare skin bore no makeup, her naked fingernails were worn short, and no jewelry adorned her body.

The professional women all stood before me in their new scrub suits, arms tightly folded against their stomachs, and tried to cover their forearms with their hands. "Aren't we allowed to wear long-sleeved covers over these?" asked Gulalai.

"No," I replied, "We have to scrub our hands up to the elbows before every birth, you know that, which means no long sleeves – not until the actual birth. Then we can put on the cover gowns." The weren't worried about blood splashing or amniotic fluid gushing onto their bare skin, otherwise they would have worried about their exposed feet in their colorful plastic sandals. They were worried about their arms. They had never exposed them in public. Ever.

"We only have one long-sleeved gown each," said Gulalai, holding it up to show me what she was talking about, "And we are accustomed to wearing this all day in our hospital. With our arms covered," she emphasized, and then translated what she'd said to her colleagues. They all nodded and frowned.

She refers to the Malalai Maternity Hospital in Kabul, where the midwives attend between 40 to 60 births every day; estimated by the Ministry of Health to be only 8% of all the births in Afghanistan. No one really knows how many babies in Afghanistan are born at home, or how many of them die, or how many women die from pregnancy-related complications or from childbirth. The last time anyone bothered to determine health statistics in Afghanistan was during the first year of the Taliban regime in 1995. In September 2002 the World Health Organization and UNICEF began coordinating thousands of local volunteers to obtain an updated survey. Most women didn't want to talk to people outside their family and less wanted to give information about their private lives, especially reproduction. The estimated maternal death ratio in Afghanistan is about 1,900 for every 100,000 births. That is to say, for every 100 babies born, two women will die. These deaths of course do not factor in a woman who died from a land mine while pregnant, or died after being beaten to death by her family for dishonor while pregnant, or from getting caught in the cross-fire during a warlord feud. For comparison, the maternal mortality ratio for Iraq (before this latest war) was only 250 per 100,000 births. In neighboring Pakistan it was 500/100,000.

At night, Muslim women are not allowed to leave their homes – in labor or not. Gulalai has lived through Russian occupation, Taliban occupation, and now American occupation – and women still do not go out at night. So she does, and always has, if she gets that phone call in the wee hours from a woman in labor who hadn't made it to the hospital during the day.

"It's what I must do," she tells me, and shrugs. Her husband, fortunately, is a rare man who feels the same way. He drives Gulalai to the women's houses, stays during the labor and birth, and shares tea with the father of the birthing woman in another part of the house.

One morning before dawn last year, coming back from an all-night labor and birth, Gulalai assumed her normal position, lying down in the back seat of the car, while her husband drove home. On that night the Taliban stopped them. They dragged them both out of the car. The Taliban men screamed at Gulalai's husband for taking his woman out at night. He said they were coming from a birth – what can they do? "No matter!" they shouted. "You know better."

They told him they would behead his wife, right there in front of him, to punish him. Gulalai's husband begged on his knees. Gulalai stood silent, her arms crossed over her chest. Finally she spoke to the these young men with rifles in a puffed up voice.

"We were at the home of Colonel Ahmed. He has a son. Go ask him." So these Taliban decided to let the couple go home, because the warlord was very famous in Kabul. However, after casually smoking the cigarettes they'd taken from Gulalai's husband, they beat him and Gulalai unconscious and left them beside their car, to show them who was the true authority here.

She told me they woke up in the morning, got into the car, and drove home. Gulalai still goes out for births. All the midwives do, even the traditional midwives, upon whom Gulalai counts for assistance where there is no one else.

Maria in Mozambique

Mozambique Fun Facts: This tropical country lies along the Indian Ocean between South Africa and Tanzania, blocking pier approval from Malawi, Zambia and Zimbabwe, which are the land-locked neighbors. Mozambique, a Portuguese colony for about 500 years, finally gained independence in 1975. It took another 30 years of in-fighting, civil war and many military rulers before relatively stable democratic elections were held in 2004. In a population estimated to be around 20 million, 1.3 million of which live with AIDS, 66% of the men can read and write while only 32% of the women can. More than half of the population is under the age of 25, with a life expectancy of just 40 years. The risk of dying of an infectious disease is very high in Mozambique, and the rate of dying while giving life (maternal mortality) is also very high; estimated by the World Health Organization to be 1,000/100,000. And for every 1,000 babies that manage to be born, 110 of them won't live past their first month.

Maria moved to the capital, Maputo, while just 16 years old in 1975 – the same year Mozambique won its independence. She emigrated with her family from the northwest Zambezi river valley during the flood season – "her family" meant herself and her six younger siblings. The "men with guns" had killed her father, mother, grandfather and older brother while she had the children gathered together in the chicken coop during the massacre. She tells me this with a straight face, as if it were just one more story of one more family. And, sadly, it is.

Maria and the siblings lived with other family members, all crammed into small and stuffy rooms over a butcher's wholesale market near the port. She worked with meat packers after school, and learned about anatomy and physiology from the animal dissection surrounding her. Today Maria proudly tells me how she also learned midwifery skills from the butcher's wife. She assisted the midwife with all the births and newborns in that area of the city where the poorest immigrants lived. "They paid us with what they had, if they had anything," said Maria. "Sometimes that meant more chickens, or fish, or scraps from the shipyards. I remember the midwife never refused any of those pieces of trash, although I never knew what she did with any of it."

Maria graduated from high school, which was a great cause for celebration in her community. The midwife and the butcher volunteered to sponsor further studies for her at the technical institute to learn nursing. Today, Maria is a well-respected, gray-haired and middle-aged nurse who is in charge of the maternity ward at the public health center. Her large hands are smooth and strong, and look like they could handle sides of beef, breech births or any obstacle in between – and they have. When she puts her palms out, spreads her fingers and declares, "Stop right there," one doesn't argue with Maria.

She tells me about the many times she had to attend births at night, and hide with the mother and newborn for the next few days while machine-gun-fire riddled the sides of the buildings near them during the years of civil war. "I always advocated breast-feeding, of course," says Maria, "But especially because having the babe at breast continuously would keep the newborn from crying and attracting the attention of those madmen. It would help keep the mother calm, also." Once, some young men did enter the room just after the mother had given birth. Maria was attending the birth of the placenta when the door burst open. The juveniles stared in silence, mouths open, guns limp at their sides. Maria stood up, put both her big hands up, palms out, fingers spread, and said, "Wait. I just have to get the placenta out. There shouldn't be that much more blood." One man fainted. The others dragged him out of the room, laughing. Mother and baby were fine. "I thought I would wet my pants just then, but I didn't. The mother squirted out that placenta and didn't bleed one more drop. I often wonder," Maria reflects with a wink in her eye, "if I should threaten more mothers with gunfire to get their placenta's out without bleeding."

There are millions of midwife stories involving gunfire and good luck, birthing amid threats of death, and perseverance in the face of perversion. Women and men continue to make love in spite of their circumstances. Men continue to rape women because of power issues. And women continue to bring life into their dying world. This scenario is played out today in many places of the world, of course: in refugee camps from Darfur to Gaza to Congo, in prostituted areas from Baltimore to Shanghai to Sao Paolo, in rural isolation from Bolivia to Mongolia to Indonesia. While men prove their manhood by destruction, disconnection and control, women risk their lives and bring a new life into the world by losing control, and connecting with anyone who is trustworthy or accessible to assist her – and in 90% of the world, that means the midwife.

*   *   *   *

Midwives around the world are inclined to emphasize relationship, links, correlation, and connection. For example, a very interesting coalition of midwives formed in 2000 from a meeting in Ceará, Brazil involving midwives and others from Mexico to Antarctica. This Latin American and Caribbean coalition has conferences, publish articles, maintains web sites, develops programs and conduct studies. They call themselves the *Red Latino Americano y Caribe para la Humanización del Parto y Nacimiento* (the Latin American & Caribbean Network for the Humanization of Childbirth), known on their web page by the acronym RELACAHUPAN [www.relacahupan.org] and they consist of more than 20 various national organizations.

These organizations have petitioned for official recognition at the United Nations, the World Bank, the World Health Organization, the International Confederation of Midwives, and the United Nations Fund for Population Development. Among their members they have traditional midwives, and have just published a Declaration for the Practice of Traditional Midwifery in the Americas. RELACAHUPAN has proposed the following Declaration:[103]

It is in our interest that any document of legislative proposal or action for the regulation of Midwifery, by the WHO or others, provide a law or regulation that is appropriate for our region and defines clearly the role of the traditional midwife. The traditional midwife should be protected with the same deference as the traditional midwife of the aboriginal communities (they are closely related). Any legislative proposal that influences our region should include:

- Written mention of the recognized name in our region: Traditional Midwife.
- Declaration of the right of the traditional midwife to maintain her profession in a manner that is respected, preserved, promoted and developed.
- Establishment in writing of the Traditional Midwife's right to be respected and recognized as primary care provider for mothers and babies in her region by other health care personnel.
- Establishment of a mechanism of close collaboration with other health professionals and provision of equipment for prevention and emergencies.
- Recognition of her natural autonomy. In any written document the word "collaboration" should be used and not the word "supervision." The interdependence should be reflected with this term.
- Regulation for the protection of providers of homebirths and for the right of mothers to be attended at home as well as the recognition that homebirth is the only option some women have.
- Establishment in writing that gifts or other bribes used by health facilities as tokens to bring

mothers away from their traditional midwives into a government health facility shall be illegal.

- Protection in favor of the traditional midwife. She shall not be offended, demoralized, or discriminated against because of age, illiteracy or other reasons; nor used in disguised or open mechanisms of elimination; and she shall not be oppressed or forced to stop or change her role, or be reduced in numbers.

One other statement tucked away inside their Declaration is this: "The development of midwifery practice in very poor areas is imperative. A change to reduce poverty and the possibility to establish health facilities in the near future is very improbable for most communities. Risk factors for poor health outcomes are related to poverty, not to the work of the traditional midwife."

Midwives probably know better than economists that poverty is the great killer of men, women, children, and newborns. Economic stability is the only sure escape from disease and indignity. How one achieves economic stability and equity depends on factors way beyond the scope of this book; suffice it to say that without nourishment, a person cannot flourish, and neither can a society.

Remember the hierarchy of needs proposed by psychiatrist Abraham Maslow back in the 1950s? He postulated that only when basic needs are met can human beings evolve to their highest achievement, which, for the purposes of his psychological health definitions, means self-actualization. The first basic need is food, and the second is security. Why, then, is a newborn baby separated from its mother at birth?

Habit based on fear by the medically trained provider can be the only excuse, because common sense and scientific evidence all point to the contrary. In order to learn to change our habits, we probably should learn about the long and tortuous history of how those habits became established and for whose benefit. Why were most midwives considered "witches?"

Pregnant Pause

The Midwife's Birth Bag

According to *Myles Textbook for Midwives* (a British midwifery text), the following items should be included in a home birth bag[104]:

- Plastic apron
- Nail brush
- Disposable sterile gloves
- Urinary test strips
- Disposable enema
- Urinary catheters
- Labour progress charts
- Birth notification forms
- Fetal stethoscope
- 2 thermometers
- Scales for baby
- Tape measurer
- Disposable mucus extractors
- Cord clamps
- Lotions: Savlon (an antiseptic)
- Alcohol swabs
- Drugs: pethidine, Naloxone (Narcan®), vitamin K, Lidocaine 1%, Ergometrine, oxytocin
- Disposable syringes and needles
- Entonox (nitrous oxide and oxygen gas)
- Bag and mask for infant resuscitation
- Baby oxygen cylinder
- Bowls
- Kidney dish for instruments
- Measuring cup for blood loss
- 2 pair cord forceps, 1 pair cord scissors
- 1 pair episiotomy scissors
- Sterile cotton balls

- Perineum pads and dressing towels
- Suture equipment

When I worked in the mountains in Bolivia and carried my birth bag with me to attend births - in a cornfield or in a bed - here is what I carried with me:

- Reading glasses (to protect from blood splash and also to read a book while I waited)
- Nail brush and disinfectant soap
- Disposable sterile gloves
- IV equipment (including 2 liters of saline and glucose formula)
- Labor progress chart
- Flashlight and extra batteries
- Granola bars and other energy foods/liquids (for me)
- Rehydration salts for making liter of rehydration solution (for her)
- Dried fruit and candies for the other kids
- Blood pressure cuff
- Stethoscopes – fetal, adult, and pediatric
- Thermometer
- Bulb syringe (mucus extractor)
- Dried herbs for teas during labor, for the placenta/postpartum, and for the sitz bath after the birth: skullcap with valerian, orange blossom, raspberry leaf, aloe vera gel, comfrey, and others
- Olive oil (for massages)
- Disposable sterile syringes/needles
- Oxytocin vial
- 1 vial ampicillin (500mg)
- Sterile gauzes
- Suturing equipment
- Cord clamps (plastic, sterile)
- Cord scissors
- Sanitary pads
- Plastic bowls
- Clean towels for the baby
- Cloth baby diaper (my gift to her)

CHAPTER 12

How are Midwives Like Witches?

Let's talk about another meaning of the word authority, which can be "power over." In *War is a Force That Gives Us Meaning*,[105] Hedges writes about the Thanatos[106] instinct that, he says, drives men toward individual and collective suicide. Hedges describes soldiers in every country he covered during his fifteen years as a war correspondent, young men who came to believe that killing is the only real form of power. "However much soldiers regret killing once it is finished," he writes, "however much they spend their lives trying to cope with the experience, the act itself, fueled by fear, excitement, the pull of peers, and the god-like exhilaration . . . is often thrilling."

Men and women know of the divine power to destroy, and this force, even if it's only potential, is rewarded and valued by every society on Earth. Men can never know the divine power to give life, and, sadly for humanity, have spent thousands of years inventing cultural constructs to get their heads around that basic fact – constructs that include religion, law, medicine, education, psychiatry, and war – to control the one thing they have no control over: human reproduction. In fact, the only physical means they have to control their own human reproduction, outside of vasectomy, is celibacy or death. Through their constructs they obviously want to control other humans' reproduction – the only "other" being women.

Women were not always thought of as property, of course. In the beginning of time, God was a woman. Think about it: for millions of years of human growth and development, before anyone connected copulation with growing a baby (because intercourse doesn't always lead to pregnancy), everyone believed that a woman controlled her ability to stop bleeding whenever she chose. That women could bleed every month without dying seemed miraculous enough, but when a woman could stay the flow of her own blood, and then grow a new human inside of her, she definitely demonstrated her divinity. She also revealed her divine capacity to feed that new life with milk from her own blood through the breasts. (Men couldn't do that either.) Blood became sacred, and women's blood the most sacred. (Think "Holy Grail" here.) The ability to spill blood for the kill reiterated that blood is the Life Force.

Additionally, all humans know who the mother is; political constructs invented by men (like the words "illegitimate" or "legitimate") instruct us who the father is. Also, ancient woman had the *power of life and death* over that helpless child for at least the first year of its life. All new human beings see a woman's face in their most holy imaginings of an all-seeing, all-powerful, all-present Supreme Being.

When men and women connected sex with babies, and when women became merely the vessel for man's magic seed, then the face of God became bearded. That belief system didn't develop overnight, nor even over the course of a few centuries. Up until the eighteenth century, medical "science" still believed that human life formed in the womb from coagulated blood. Changing the face of God from woman to man took forethought and malice, cunning and ingenuity, great planning and great care over several centuries – the results of which have had devastating effects on our environment, our societies, and our health ever since. There are many interesting anthropological, archeological and sociological books written on the subject of subjugation in all cultures from China to Chad, Latvia to Latin America, Afghanistan to Australia, and detailing those histories would be beyond the scope of this book.

However, allow me a quick review of more recent world history; let's go over the Burning Times as just one brutal example of how patriarchal passion forced people to believe the face of God was male. Oh, dear. Didn't you study that in your high school World History class?

Me neither. You may have been exposed to a paragraph or two that mentioned the "Dark Ages," or that many women were burned at the stake for being "witches." You may have even learned that the Inquisition was instigated by the Catholic Church to rid the world of "devil worshippers" – unless you attended Catholic High School. What you may not have known about the trials of these women, girls, grandmothers, widows, and maiden aunts is that all the judges were men (even though some of the accusers were women). And the majority of those judges were doctors. And the majority of the properties of those women were confiscated by the Church. And the majority of those who were sentenced to be doused in oil and burned alive in front of their children or tortured in other hideous ways until dead were midwives.

Consider the following statistics, taken from meticulously documented pages of judges and inquisitors:[107]

- "Witch hunting" began around the early 1300s and lasted about *400 years* in most European countries and in the New World (northern and southern hemispheres).
- The most popular document legalizing this mass murder, titled *Malleus Maleficarum*, or the Witches' Hammer, was written in 1486 by the German Dominican inquisitors Heinrich Kramer and Jacob Sprenger. Their working sub-title: "Because superstition is found, above all, in women."
- The text was copied from the works of Catholic priests from the years 1376 (*Directorium Inquisitorum)* and 1435 (*Formicarius*), whose

subtitles recorded, "There is no greater threat to the Catholic Church than the midwife."

- The judicial handbook *Malleus Maleficarum* was mandated by Pope Innocent VII in his Papal Bull *Summis desiderantes affectibus* and was used as a judgmental guide throughout Europe for about 300 years.
- Anyone who sided with the woman during her "trial" was also tortured or threatened with excommunication by the Christian Church (both Catholic and Protestant).
- Between 1490 and 1520, more than 600 women in Western Europe were murdered per year; about two per day for thirty years.
- 900 women were killed in only one year in Wertzberg, Germany.
- 400 were burned alive in just one day in Toulouse, France.
- In Trier in 1585, two villages were left with only two women each.
- Switzerland: 4000 people were killed of a total population of about one million (four per thousand).
- Historians estimate about 40,000 executions over 250 years in Europe, which had a population of approximately 150 million at the time with a life expectancy of about 40 years.

Even if we assume only one execution for witchcraft per 25,000 deaths, this killing spree still ranks about 3.5 times higher as a cause of death than death by capital punishment (for any offense) in the U.S. in the late 20th century. The term Dark Ages resonates for us still today.

Who were these women and what were they doing? Women became the scapegoats for misfortune, plain and simple. Psychologist Jeanne Achterberg notes that assigning blame to others yields a sense of prediction and control over our own life.[108] Witches were blamed for men's impotence, according to theologian Thomas Aquinas. These and other accusations (she wouldn't accept sexual advances, she wanted payment for her work, she rejected him, she wants that man for a husband, not this one...) proved to be a handy way to rid oneself of meddlesome wives, nagging girlfriends, rebellious adolescent daughters, or needy mothers-in-law. Most older women, living on the fringes of a male-valued society that deemed them as surplus, had to find a way to feed themselves and often used their knowledge of plants and life experiences to heal people or attend women in labor. Midwifery and folk healing were alternatives to starving. If the patient grew sick or died, the old woman was blamed. If the patient got well and healed without the (male) doctor's intervention, she was blamed for that, too.

Not only were wise women accused of healing without having studied (although they were not allowed to study, and the Catholic Church dictated exactly what could be studied in medicine for more than 800 years), they were also charged with the ability for "laying on cures and laying them off."[109] The Dominican Johann Herolt said, "Most women belie their Catholic faith with charms and spells, after the fashion of Eve...Any woman by herself knows more of such superstitions and charms than a hundred men."[110] Superstitions, charms, and spells, of course, constituted all forms of medical practice of the day.

There are countless stories of wise women during this period – women from upper, middle, and lower socio-economic classes – who attended the sick, healed the wounded, stayed with women during childbirth and afterward, cared for the dying, and generally helped out of compassion. Alison Peirsoun of Bytehill, for example, had established her reputation as a gifted healer in England. The archbishop of St. Andrew sent for her because he said he was "afflicted with many disorders" (what we would call psychosomatic today). He had been treated by many practitioners without relief. Alison, by whatever means, cured him. Later, he not only refused to pay her, he also had her arrested. She was charged and executed for witchcraft.

All these "witch" activities added to the superstitious fears of King James of England, who (probably with reason) believed that many were plotting to kill him and overthrow the kingdom. This is the same James who commissioned the first translation of the Bible from Hebrew to English (the King James version), where the word "witch" appears for the first time. (In the original Hebrew it is translated as "whisperer of spells."[111]) The most quoted passage from that Bible during the Burning Times was Exodus 22:18: "Thou shalt not suffer a witch to live."

The murder of women and some men who believed in and protected women, particularly women healers and midwives, reflects the deepest fear of women's power.[112] Belief systems that create magic and religion disturb the powerful because this intervention in times of stress relieves anxiety and gives the powerless some sense of control over uncontrollable events. The contemporary Scottish sociologist and expert on the Burning Times, Christine Larner, writes:

> The healer is a source of hope in the community. But her power is two-edged. If she should fail, demand extortionate and uneconomic returns for her services or become hostile, then she becomes a source of menace and focus for anxiety. The refusal of Canon Law to distinguish between black and white magic, while based on the idea that all power not sanctioned by the church is either ineffectual or demonic, regardless of whether it is intended to heal or harm, in fact reflects a peasant reality: that the healer can be dangerous.[113]

In her book *Woman as Healer*, Achterberg writes about how religion is joined with health and always has been. "Healing and the sacred are yoked together with the thickest of cords in the human psyche – a connection so stable that all advances in medicine, all the training to the contrary, cannot dislodge one from the other." From the earliest known cultures to the present day, how many people believe their health or illness is controlled by an unseen hand, and how many believe that the doctor is "God"? How many doctors believe they are "God"? And how many believe that having "power-over" others is the same as owning the force to cure or kill?

The healer represents power at one continuum that ends with the most abstract level: God and the Devil. During those four hundred years of sanctioned femicide, women healers were edged out of guilds (any group of like-minded individuals who form a closed society for its members), and then kept out by the incorporation of (literally "to make a body of") physicians, surgeons, and apothecaries. Women healers were prohibited by law in every country in Europe for nearly a millennium. Both the Inquisition and Christian theology had been used to exclude women from studying, from practicing, and from teaching anything that had to do with healing.

Gradually, the sanctioned murder of women during the Dark Ages phased out of fashion – not because of a change in religious beliefs, but because the Church lost its stranglehold on the governments of Europe. When religious affairs became separated from government, public nature and the sheer volume of murders diminished due to this shift and thus drew less attention...yet continued more quietly. Despite this reduction in outright femicide, women were still not allowed citizenship in any country, nor the right to own property or money or business. Those particular four hundred years of persecution served to cement the status of women to that of barely human – the definition of "human" based on male criteria – and to increase the social and practical acceptance of misogyny and distrust.

Even today, it appears that sexual obsession is central to the concept of masculinity. Robin Morgan writes about the psychological and political roots of terrorism when she describes the Taliban in her book *The Demon Lover*: "If being a man is defined as *not* being a woman, then a man must either keep separate from women (celibacy) or enslave them (mastery)."[114] Think of all the rituals and religious instruction surrounding women that have been written (by men) in their holy books: Torah, the Quran, and the Bible.

This is not a theological treatise, and there have been plenty of good books written by women (and men) about this very subject over many years. What I want to connect for us here concerns childbirth and ritual – whether that ritual is based on myths from religious texts or myths from medical texts – and how these myths perpetuate the concept of power and authority as something to be valued. These concepts do not serve us as creators and sustainers of the human race and of society; they do not serve any of us.

Why, then, do we perpetuate these myths by going along with a structure that disrespects us or denies our inner authoritative knowledge? It may be because we don't know about the tools we need in order to look for another way of being. Fortunately, we don't have to look very far. Many, many women (and men) healers are involved right now in ways to help us grow toward connection, compassion, and healing within ourselves and for healing our planet. Some may call this "New Age" or "Holistic Health." I call it common sense, and so did my grandmother, a traditional midwife.

And this is what is called for in our policies and our practices: common sense: policies and practices that favor prevention, contraception, nutrition and sanitation; policies and practices that have priority over economic incentives, convenience, and ego-stroking; policies and practices that convey cost-effectiveness along with connections – for the future of our society depends on them.

CHAPTER 13

Are We There Yet?

How am I, one person with good intentions, going to change the world? Jan Tritten, midwife and editor of *Midwifery Today* magazine, responds to that question like all midwives do: One baby at a time. How can one conscious and conscientious health care provider make a difference against the great tide of fear and habit pervading the entire medical machine that dictates how and when mothers give birth? Michel Odent, obstetrician and founder of the Primal Health Institute in London, responds to that question like all concerned physicians do: Knowledge can induce awareness, and with awareness we have hope. Thus, we can all help by disseminating knowledge – one mother, one doctor, one health care policy maker at a time.

As I mentioned in Chapter 1, those of us who have a university education think we know what's best for those who don't. Those of us raised within a certain class system believe we know what The Other needs to have a better life – like ours. Organizations and governments with their own agendas and monies are writing health care reform policy for people who have neither. Fortunately, for everyone who can read, policy can now be based on well-designed research instead of habit and fear. And although we may now have scientific evidence to show which practices are safer and why, which ones are unnecessary and why, and which ones are downright harmful, we also need to understand the nature of Nature.

In his latest book, *Creating Your Birth Plan*, [115] Dr. Marsden Wagner writes, "Childbirth hasn't changed since the beginning of history, only our attitudes and our methods [have changed]." Those attitudes and methods have at their foundation the desire to "fool Mother Nature" or to control what is inherently an out-of-control situation. Don't forget: in spite of sending men to the moon and discovering the secrets of DNA, scientists still have not discovered what makes labor start. That's right; no one knows what makes a woman's uterus begin the process of pushing the baby down into the pelvis, through the cervix, and out the vagina. Scientists have, of course, determined how it works, but not exactly what sparks that miraculous progression toward the light.

Ina May Gaskin, midwife and mentor at many births, writes in her book *Spiritual Midwifery*[116] that the way women are treated during childbirth affects them in all their relationships for the rest of their lives. The way babies are treated at birth is likely to affect them for the rest of their lives and to affect society as well. Ask your grandmother or great aunt to tell you about the birth of her child so many years ago. If she wasn't drugged at the time, she will remember every detail.

And don't forget: it is difficult for any human being to express compassion who has not learned compassion from a very early age. Compassion is not just a "nice thing" to demonstrate during the birth of a child – it lies at the very heart of a sane society. "Kindness begets kindness," says Ina May, "that is passed on to nursing babies and to proud fathers, to brothers and sisters, cousins, aunts and uncles."

Compassion is not on the curriculum at many nursing or medical schools; or if it is, you'll see it inserted in the course for the care of dying patients. Compassion takes time, and time is of the essence if we have twenty patients "to deliver" by the end of our shift (or we'll have to "deliver" them to the oncoming shift – and our peers won't like that!).

It is difficult for me to understand why women put up with this mismanagement, why they endure an open ward in a hospital to labor among strangers, why they entrust their own bodies to another person. I very much doubt that men would consent to this type of treatment. The old feminist saying may apply: If men could get pregnant, abortion would be a sacrament. How many men would expose their genitals to other men, let alone other women, even if those women were doctors? Why do women accept this bad behavior on the part of "providers"? Because we have been trained from a very young age to believe we are worth less than men, and to believe in an authority outside our Selves – the father, the doctor, the priest, the police, the God.

Here is what I have observed in every public hospital in every developing country that I have visited over the past fifteen years. After I have the obligatory political meetings with the hospital directors in their well-appointed offices, we take tea, which is served by a nurse who is thereby unavailable for patient care. As soon as we begin our obligatory guided tour of the hospital, we see the cleanest areas first, where staff are prepared to receive us. I smile graciously. I respond to demonstrations politely. I always ask the unexpected: Where is the antiseptic soap for hand washing? What happens to the used needle container once it's full? Where is the incinerator? They respond to the questions politely. They smile tightly.

As we continue our scrutiny into the labor ward, we see the worst area of every hospital, where doors remain open to exposed women. Because our WHO-mandated hospital evaluations are obligatory templates for all cultures in every country, we see similarities that show every hospital administrator's office to be more beautiful than any labor and delivery ward, which is unequipped to serve tea.

The administrators are always doctors, and they are almost always men. Many will use the excuse that they have no budget for private birthing rooms. Many more will say they have no room to build even if they did have the budget, or no staff, or no contracts, or no reason to build private rooms. Is it any wonder that the women who do have sufficient self-respect and autonomy choose home birth over hospital birth in developing countries? And that the majority choose to be attended by traditional midwives?

Many doctors will argue that these same women are the ones dying by the truckload and need to come into a health care facility in order to be helped by professionals who can save their lives and the lives of their babies. Some countries even offer free prenatal and childbirth care in their public hospitals. "Come to us!" they cry, standing at the hospital door in their white, starched lab coats with their shiny stethoscopes around their white-collared necks. "We will save you!" Many, many women in many, many countries have told me, "I would rather die in my home than have that doctor expose me, humiliate me, cut me, or take my baby from me."

And even after many studies showing us that women (and their husbands) value human respect over cold, hard statistics, men (and women) of science continue to insist that women come into those barbaric places to give birth. Even when they are convinced to accept this condemnation, women are never happy about their decision afterward. "It's something I just had to do for my mother-in-law," say many women. "My husband wanted us to be safe," say many others, with a sigh and a caveat: "At least I have a healthy baby."

But don't forget: scientific evidence[117] shows that *more women die from hospital births than from a planned home birth;* many more babies die in hospitals than at home; and induced labor leads to higher cesarean section operations – from which more women die than from vaginal childbirth. Health policy planners and physicians will counter that many more women in developing countries die at home during childbirth or during the postpartum period than at hospitals, but they are wrong. There are entire books written about that error of thinking, including two involved with health policy.[118]

A childbearing woman faces death every time she becomes pregnant – that's nature, and she knows it. The ones who die usually do so from hemorrhage, bleeding to death because they don't have enough red blood cells with clotting factors. They don't have enough red blood cells because they are malnourished, or they have suffered from malaria, or because they have had untreated infections, or, if they live in the United States, because they were murdered. As we saw in Chapter Three, the definitions of maternal mortality don't often tell the whole story; for instance, the story of poverty that leads up to a hemorrhage, of an enraged boyfriend that leads to murder, or of religious restrictions that lead to unsafe and illegal abortion. And we are just talking about the mother. What happens to all those babies who die within days of being born?

"Most neonatal deaths occur at home, following unsupervised deliveries," write the doctors from the World Health Organization in their book about how to improve birth outcomes in developing countries.[119] The very next sentence says that because most births in the world occur at home, there is very little, if any, accurate information about the cause of death! They go on to speculate that the majority of babies die of birth asphyxia – not breathing at birth. This is just a handy way to blame the victims: mothers and fathers rarely have had classes on newborn resuscitation. Traditional midwives are not taught this easy skill, either. They are taught to "transport the baby to the health facility" where, supposedly, someone will be on call who knows how to resuscitate a deceased newborn, hours after the birth.

The fact is that most babies die at home in undeveloped countries because they were born underweight to malnourished mothers, or to mothers who had malaria, AIDS, tuberculosis, or other infectious diseases that went untreated. Some babies die from exposure, a time-honored family planning method for thousands of years in undeveloped countries where pregnancies are not wanted, husbands make health policy, and contraceptives don't exist.

What about countries with very good nutrition, with well-staffed hospitals and highly trained personnel and women who are convinced that abdominal surgery is a better way to birth their baby? Why do countries like Chile, Israel, or the UK still have maternal mortality rates above their neighboring countries?[120] Why does the richest country in the world (as of this writing, the U.S.) have maternal mortality rates higher than Serbia and Montenegro – two countries barely out of a deadly civil war? Is it the way these deaths are counted?

Women are worthy. Women who give birth are worthy of the best our society has to offer them – including resources, good nutrition, clean water, a safe environment, and respect. Women who attend these women are worthy of the highest social regard and remuneration. Why does a common soldier, who kills other humans, earn more money per month than a midwife who helps women bring new life into the world? Apparently because death is a force that gives many people meaning. Fear is a powerful engine that drives many social, medical, and public health programs.

We know that evidence, education, and information can and does help to eradicate fear. We know that women who respect themselves and who demand respect from others have the highest health and educational statistics in every country. We know that love is a powerful force that delivers us from evil. If childbirth were allowed to happen in an atmosphere of love and respect, then we could truly know, in the depths of our being, that birth is a force that gives all of us meaning.

Pregnant Pause

Ain't I a Woman?
Sojourner Truth, 1797-1883

That man over there say
a woman needs to be helped into carriages
and lifted over ditches
and to have the best place everywhere.
Nobody ever helped me into carriages or over mud puddles
or gives me a best place...
And ain't I a woman?

Look at me
Look at my arm!
I have plowed and planted
and gathered into barns
and no man could head me...
And ain't I a woman?
I could work as much
and eat as much as a man—
when I could get to it—
and bear the lash as well
and ain't I a woman?

I have born 13 children
and seen most all sold into slavery
and when I cried out a mother's grief
none but Jesus heard me...
and ain't I a woman?

That little man in black there say
a woman can't have as much rights as a man
cause Christ wasn't a woman

Where did your Christ come from?
From God and a woman!
Man had nothing to do with him!

If the first woman God ever made was strong enough
to turn the world upside down,
all alone,
then together women ought to be able
to turn it right-side up again.

A few Web sites for more information - get involved!

- http://www.thewhiteribbonalliance.org
- http://www.childbirthconnection.org
- http://www.imbci.org/
- http://www.news-medical.net/news/17442.aspx
- http://www.midwifeinfo.com/
- http://www.motherfriendly.org/
- http://www.birthinternational.com/index.html
- http://partera.com/pages_en/tpe.html
- http://www.internationalmidwives.org
- http://mana.org/
- http://devex.com/signups/healthcare?gclid=CMKIo5T
St5oCFRSfnAodVCNUcQ
- http://www.usaid.gov/our_work/global_health/mch/
index.html
- http://www.dfid.gov.uk/
- http://www.deutsche-kultur-international.de/en/org/
organizations/german-organisation-for-technial-coop-
eration-gtz.html
- http://www.who.int/reproductive-health/publications/
maternal_mortality_2005/mme_2005.pdf
- http://www.who.int/publications/en/
- http://www.who.int/whosis/whostat/2008/en/index.
html
- http://www.who.int/reproductive-health/MNBH/in-
dex.htm
- http://www.birthworks.org/site/primal-health-re-
search.html

References

[1] Hedges, C. 2002, *War is a Force That Gives Us Meaning*, Anchor Books, NY

[2] Rook, J.P. 1997, *Midwifery & Childbirth in America*, Temple University Press, Philadelphia

[3] Martin, E. 1992, *The Woman in the Body: A cultural analysis of reproduction*, Beacon Press, Boston

[4] http://www.who.int/reproductive-health/publications/maternal_mortality_2000/index.html

[5] Editorial in *The Boston Globe*, "Violence Against Women," December 8, 2006

[6] Wagner, M. 1994, *Pursuing the Birth Machine – The search for appropriate birth technology*, ACE Graphics, Australia

[7] Cunningham, McDonald and Gant, 1989, *Williams Obstetrics*, Appleton & Lange, Connecticut

[8] Gaskin, I. 1978, *Spiritual Midwifery*, The Farm Book Press, Summertown, TN, USA

[9] Davis-Floyd, R. 1992, *Birth as an American Rite of Passage*, University of California Press.

[10] Richmond, J. 1990, Keynote address at the American Academy of Pediatrics Conference on Cross-national Comparisons of Child Health, Washington, D.C., March 1990

[11] See their training programs at www.jhpiego.net

[12] Andreason, A. 1995, *Marketing Social Change – Changing Behavior to Promote Health, Social Development, and the Environment*, Jossey-Bass Press, Washington, D.C.

[13] Paluzzi, J. 2004, *Primary Health Care Since Alma Ata – Lost in the Breton Woods?* Chapter 4 in *Unhealthy Health Policy – A critical anthropological examination*, Castro and Singer, eds., Alta Mira Press, New York, NY

[14] *Revised 2000 Estimates of Maternal Mortality: a WHO and UNICEF review;* WHO, Geneva. 2005 www.who.int/reproductive-health/publications/maternal_ mortality_2000/maternal_mortality_2000.pdf

15 www.segeplan.gob.gt/ine/index.htm

16 Child Maltreat. 2003 May;8(2):122-8; Krulewitch, C. Adolescent pregnancy and homicide: Findings from the Maryland office of the chief medical examiner, 1994-1998

17 www.who.int/bookorders/anglais/detart1.jsp?sesslan=1&codlan=1&codcol=15&codcch=1592

18 JAMA. 2001 Mar 21;285(11):1510-1; Frye, V. Editorial: Examining homicide's contribution to pregnancy-associated deaths

19 http://www.reproductive-health-journal.com/content/2/1/3#IDAHI2YL

20 www.who.int/entity/mediacentre/news/releases/2004/pr65/en/

21 Pizarro, A. Women's Health in Nicaragua: The need for a secular state; IRC America's Program, Mar 2004 at www.americas.irc-online.org/reports/2004/0403nicawom.html

22 Pizarro, ibid.

23 The Guttmacher Report on Public Policy, May 2003, Volume 6, Number 2; Envisioning Life Without Roe: Lessons Without Borders; Cohen, S.

24 http://whqlibdoc.who.int/publications/2004/9241591838.pdf

25 womanway@aol.com and www.midwivesformidwives.com for more information about the Midwives for Midwives organization

26 See their web sites for more information: http://www.mana.org/ and http://www.iam.org and for more definitions see http://www.mana.org/definitions.html#MMOC

27 Ibid.

28 Benoit, C. 2002, "An Exception to the Canadian Case: Autonomous Midwifery at the Margins" in *Midwifery and the Medicalization of Childbirth – Comparative perspectives*; Ed. Van Teijlingen et. al. Nova Sciences Publishers, Inc.

29 Safe Motherhood Policy Alert, No.4, Nov 2003; *The Kenya Safe Motherhood Demonstration Project*; Kenya Ministry of Health, the University of Nairobi, and the Population Council.

30 *Curationis*, 1997 Mar;20(1):15-20 "The Importance of Traditional Midwives in the Delivery of Health Care in the Republic of South Africa;" Troskie, T.R.

31 Carrasco, M. 2000, Poetas mapuches en la literatura chilena; *Estudios Filológicos,* No. 35; Universidad Austral de Chile, Valdivia, Chile

32 Ministerio de Salud de Chile, Programa de la Mujer, 2000.

33 Davis-Floyd, R. 1992, op. cit.

34 Jordan, B. 1983, *Birth in Four Cultures,* Eden Press, Ontario, Canada.

35 Vidales, A. 2006, *Políticas Económicas Aplicadas a la Salud,* Universidad de Valparaíso, Chile

36 Editorial, *Journal of the American Medical Association,* 44 (1905); p. 1933

37 Achterberg, Jeanne, 1991, *Woman as Healer,* Shambhala Press, London

38 Ibid.

39 https://www.cia.gov/cia/publications/factbook/geos/id.html#Govt

40 Achadi, E. et.al. 2000, *The MotherCare Experience in Indonesia – Final Report,* John Snow, Inc. Arlington, VA

41 http://www.kalimantan.com/s/Home.asp

42 Achadi, E. et.al. 2000, op. cit.

43 Ibid.

44 Program Brief: Preventing Postpartum Hemorrhage – A community based approach proves effective in rural Indonesia, 2000, JHPIEGO, an affiliate of The Johns Hopkins University, Baltimore Maryland, USA

45 Lars Høj, et.al. 2005. Effect of sublingual misoprostol on severe postpartum haemorrhage in a primary health centre in Guinea-Bissau: randomised double blind clinical trial. *British Medical Journal,* October 1; 331(7519): 723. Also: El-Refaey H., et al. 2000. The misoprostol third stage of labor study: A randomised controlled comparison trial between orally administered misoprostol and standard management. *The British Journal of Obstetrics and Gynaecology*: 107: 1104–1110; McCormick, M.L., et al. 2002, Preventing postpartum hemorrhage in low-resource settings. *International Journal of Obstetrics and Gynecology*; 77(3): 267–275; and Ng PS et al. 2001. A multicentre randomized controlled trial of oral misoprostol

and intramuscular syntometrine in the management of the third stage of labour. *Human Reproduction*; 16(1): 31–35.

46   Program Brief: Preventing Postpartum Hemorrhage, op. cit.

47   Lars Høj, et.al. 2005, op. cit.

48   http://en.wikipedia.org/wiki/Prostaglandins

49   Emily Westheimer, and Jennifer Blum, 2003, Misoprostol – A new addition to post abortion care, Gyunity Health Projects, New York. http:/www.gynuity.org/documents/miso_pac_mtg_1003.pdf

50   Ibid.

51   Beech, B. 2006, Misoprostol for Induction of Labour: Untested, Unapproved and Unnecessary. *Association for Improvements in the Maternity Services Journal*; Autumn 2001;13(3) Also: http://www.aims.org.uk/Journal/Vol13No3/misoprostol1.htm

52   Alfirevic Z, Weeks A. "Oral Misoprostol for Induction of Labour," *The Cochrane Database of Systematic Reviews* 2006 Issue 4; also http://www.cochrane.org/reviews/en/ab001338.html

53   Goer, H. The Assault on Normal Birth – The OB Disinformation Campaign in *Midwifery Today*; (63) Autumn 2003

54   Goldberg, A. B., Greenberg, B.S., & Darney, P. D. 2001, Misoprostol and pregnancy, *N Engl J Med* 344: 38-47

55   Federal Drug Administration web site www.fda.gov/medwatch/SAFETY/2002/safety02.htm#cytote

56   Reuters: FDA OKs label change for labor-inducing drug. Reuters Health Information, Apr 18, 2002

57   Goer, H. 1995, *Obstetric Myths versus Research Realities – A guide to the medical literature*, Bergin & Garvey, London, page 185 for list of studies

58   Otto, C and Platt, LD. Fetal Growth and Development, *Obstet Gynecol Clin North Am* 1991; 18(4):907 - 931

59   Olesen, AW and Thomsen, SG, Prediction of Delivery Date in the First and Second Trimesters, *Ultrasound Obstet Gynecol*; 2006 Sep;28(3):292-7

60   Cesario, SK, Re-evaluation of Friedman's Labor Curve, *J Obstet Gynecol Neonatal Nurs* 2004 Nov- Dec;33(6):713-22.

61 Cecilia, Carmen, and Tía Susie are invented names to protect the women's privacy. All other names and all the events are true.

62 http://americas.irc-online.org/reports/2004/0403nicawom.html

63 Ibid.

64 N.C. Aizenman, "Nicaragua's Total Ban On Abortion Spurs Critics," article in *The Washington Post*, November 28, 2006

65 Ibid.

66 http://www.radiofeminista.net/nov06/notas/observatorio_audios.htm

67 http://americas.irc-online.org/reports/2004/0403nicawom.html

68 Achterberg, J. 1991, op. cit.

69 For an interesting explanation of medical anthropology see the Society for Medical Anthropology web site at http://www.medanthro.net/definition.html

70 Davis-Floyd, R. and Sargent, C. eds., 1997, *Childbirth and Authoritative Knowledge – Cross cultural perspectives*, University of California Press

71 Lightfoot-Klein, H. *Erroneous Belief Systems Underlying Female Genital Mutilation in Sub-Saharan Africa and Male Neonatal Circumcision in the United States*, presentation at Third Annual Symposium on Circumcision, University of Maryland, College Park, MD; 1994; also http://www.nocirc.org/symposia/third/hanny3.html

72 Ibid.

73 Grimes, R. 2000, *Deeply Into the Bone – Re-inventing rites of passage*; University of California Press

74 Davis-Floyd, R. 1992, op. cit.

75 For clarification on the difference between technocratic vs. holistic models of birth, see "Pregnant Pause" on page 67.

76 Kitzinger, S. 2000, *Rediscovering Birth*; Pocket Books, London.

77 Lewis, M. Giving Birth in Berkeley – The father's perspective, *Slate Magazine*, Monday, Jan 8, 2007.

78 Hedges, C. 2002, op. cit.

79 Taylor, S. E., Klein, et.al. "Female Responses to Stress: Tend and Befriend, Not Fight or Flight," *Psychological Review*; 2000. 107(3),41-429.

80 Berkowitz, G. "UCLA Study on Friendship Among Women" in *Postpartum Support International* at http://www.postpartum. net/friendship.html

81 Kitzinger, S. Ibid.

82 Kroeger, M. and Pascali-Bonaro, D. "Continuous female companionship during childbirth: a crucial resource in times of stress or calm," *Journal of Midwifery and Women's Health*; 2004. Jul-Aug;49(4) Supplement 1:19-27

83 Hodnett, E. 1995, "Support from Caregivers During Childbirth" in *Pregnancy and Childbirth Module of Cochrane Database of Systemic Reviews*, BMJ, London.

84 Ablow, K. "The Perilous Journey from Delivery Room to Bedroom" in *The New York Times*, Aug 23, 2005.

85 Ibid.

86 Kitzinger, S. 2000, op. cit.

87 See article online by Kitzinger in *Birth* (Blackwell Publishing), "The Clock, The Bed and The Chair." http://www.sheilakitzinger. com/ArticlesBySheila/BIRTH_March2003.htm

88 For more information, see http://maternidadlaluz.com/index. sstg

89 Russell, J. ed., 2001, The Maternal Brain: neurobiological and neuroendocrine adaptation and disorders in pregnancy and postpartum. In *Progress in Brain Research* (Vol 133) Elsevier Press.

90 Davis-Floyd, R. 1992, op. cit.

91 Myhran, A. et.al. 1996, Unwantedness of a pregnancy and schizophrenia of a child. *British Journal of Psychiatry*. 169:637-640

92 Odent, M. 1999, *The Scientification of Love*, Free Association Books, London

93 Raine, A, et.al. Birth Complications combined with early maternal rejection at age one year predispose to violent crimes at 18 years. *Arch Gen Psychiatry* 1994;51:984-8

94 Jacobson, B. and Nyberg, K. Opiate addiction in adult offspring through possible imprinting after obstetric treatment. *British Medical Journal* 1998;317; 1346-9

95 Hattori, R. et al. Autistic and developmental disorders after general anesthetic delivery. *Lancet* June 1991; 337; 1357-8

96 Modahl Charlotte, Green LA, Fein D, Morris M, Waterhouse L, Feinstein C, et al. Plasma oxytocin levels in autistic children. *Biol Psychiatry* 1998;43(4):270– 7.

97 Green L, Fein D, Modahl C, Feinstein C, Waterhouse L, Morris M. Oxytocin and autistic disorder: alterations in peptide forms. *Biol Psychiatry* 2001;50:609– 13.

98 Carter CS. The neuroendocrinology of social attachment and love. *Psychoneuroendocrinology* 1998; 23:779– 818.

99 MacFarlane, J.A. 1975. Olfaction in the development of social preference in the human neonate. In *The Human Neonate in Parent-Infant Interaction* pages 103-117; Ciba Foundation Symposium 33; Amsterdam. Elsevier Press, Oxford

100 Ferguson, J. et.al. Social amnesia in mice lacking the oxytocin gene. *Nature Genetics* Jul 2000; 25:3;284-288

101 Moss, I.R. et.al. 1982. Human beta endorphin-like immuno-reactivity in the perinatal and neonatal period. *J of Pediatrics* 101(3):443-446

102 All Fun Facts introducing each of the true stories come from the World Health Organization document *Maternal Mortality in 2000: Estimates Developed by WHO, UNICEF and UNFPA* by Carla AbouZahra and Tessa Wardlawa; and from the CIA web site www.cia.gov/cia

103 "The Traditional Midwife in Our Region" Declaration to the International Confederation of Midwives, the International Federation of Gynecologists and Obstetricians, the World Health Organization and the World Bank, March 2007, RELACAHUPAN web site www.relacahupan.org

104 Bennett, V. Ruth and Linda K. Brown, eds. 1989, *Myles Textbook for Midwives*, eleventh edition, Churchill Livingstone Press, London [This was written before AIDS precautions were universally recommended.]

105 Hedges, C. 2002, op. cit.

106 In Freudian psychoanalytic theory, Thanatos [from the Greek myths] is sometimes used to refer to the death drive because it is opposed to Eros, the life drive. In Freud's theory, Eros is characterized as the tendency towards cohesion and unity, whereas the death drive is the tendency towards destruction.

107 Quotations from the list are from the following sources:
  Woman As Healer by Jeanne Achterberg, 1991, Shambhala Press, London
  Witches, Midwives and Nurses – History of Women Healers by Ehrenreich and English, 1973, Feminist Press, NY
  Adam, Eve and the Serpent by Elaine Pagels, 1988, Vintage Books, New York
  The Woman's Encyclopedia of Myths and Secrets by Barbara Walker, 1983, Harper Collins, NY

108 Jeanne Achterberg, 1991, op. cit.

109 Ibid.

110 V. Bullough, 1973, *The Subordinate Sex*, University of Chicago Press

111 Many thanks to personal correspondence for these and other Biblical clarifications from Maryl Smith, Certified Professional Midwife and Theology major who may be contacted at http://www.worshipwithoutborders.org/index.php?s=about#maryl

112 Jeanne Achterberg, 1991, op. cit.

113 Larner, C. 1981, *Enemies of God*, Johns Hopkins University Press, Baltimore

114 Morgan, R. 2001, *The Demon Lover – The Roots of Terrorism*; Washington Square Press, New York

115 Wagner, M. with Stephanie Gunning, 2006, *Creating Your Birth Plan – The definitive guide to a safe and empowering birth*; Penguin Books, NY

116 Gaskin, Ina May, 1990, op. cit.

117 Any remaining doubts about the safety of home birth were conclusively erased by the publication of a very large, scientifically rigorous study of more than 5,000 planned home birth with midwives. K. Johnson and B. Daviss, Outcomes of Planned Home Births with Certified Professional Midwives:

Large prospective study in North America. *British Medical Journal* 330 (June 2005): 1416.

[118] Castro, A. and Singer, M. eds. 2004, *Unhealthy Health Policy – A critical anthropological examination*, Altamira Press, Walnut Creek, California and The Institute of Medicine; 2003 *Improving Birth Outcomes – Meeting the challenge in the developing world*, The National Academies Press, Washington DC

[119] Ibid.

[120] All the statistics with explanations about MMR can be found in the 2004 WHO document *Maternal Mortality in 2000: Estimates developed by WHO, UNICEF, UNFPA*; Department of Reproductive Health and Research World Health Organization, Geneva or at
http://www.who.int/reproductivehealth/publications/maternal_mortality_2000/mme.pdf